AORTIC ANEURYSM

Edited by **Kaan Kırali**

Aortic Aneurysm
http://dx.doi.org/10.5772/62928
Edited by Kaan Kırali

Contributors

Deniz Günay, Kaan Kırali, Yasir Alsiraj, Sean Thatcher, Cassis, Ibrahim Akin, Alex Sher, Rami Tadros, Katarzyna Stefańczyk, Ludomir Stefańczyk, Michał Polguj, Ting-Wei Lin, Chung-Dann Kan, Idit Avrahami, Ismail Cassimjee, Regent Lee, Jyoti Patel, Hila Ben Gur, Gabor Kosa, Saar Golan, Moshe Brand

Published by InTech
Janeza Trdine 9, 51000 Rijeka, Croatia

Publishing Process Manager Iva Simcic
Technical Editor SPi Global
Cover InTech Design team

First published February, 2017
Printed in Croatia
Legal deposit, Croatia: National and University Library in Zagreb

Additional hard copies can be obtained from orders@intechopen.com

Aortic Aneurysm, Edited by Kaan Kırali
p. cm.
Print ISBN 978-953-51-2933-2
Online ISBN 978-953-51-2934-9

For EU product safety concerns:
IN TECH d.o.o., Prolaz Marije Krucifikse Kozulić 3, 51000 Rijeka, Croatia,
info@intechopen.com or visit our website at intechopen.com.

Meet the editor

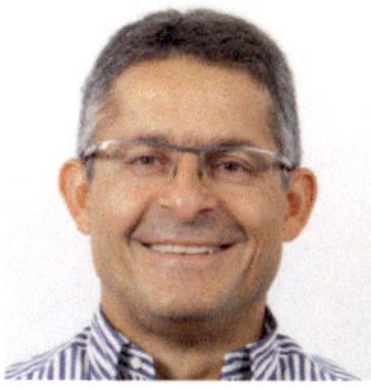

With a medical degree in Turkey, upon his cardiovascular PhD degree in 1997 at Kosuyolu Heart and Research Hospital in Istanbul, Prof. Kırali is codetermining two cardiac centers: head of Heart Transplantation and Mechanical Support Department of Kosuyolu Hospital (Istanbul) and CVS Department of the Faculty of Medicine of Sakarya University (Sakarya). Over the last 20 years, he has focused his scientific interests on the topics related to cardiovascular therapies requiring experience. With his expertise in coronary bypass surgery, minimal invasive cardiac surgery, vascular surgery, and aortic root surgery, he has been interested in aortic valve-sparing operations in the last years. He has developed a new aortotomy technique, surgical approaches for calcific aortic stenosis, and complication-free stentless and sutureless aortic valve replacement procedures. He has also been interested in the above preventive medicine since his public health MHSc degree in 2000 at Istanbul University. He published numerous SCI journal papers and book chapters and edited/reviewed many academic journals.

Contents

Preface

Aortic aneurysm is a life-threatening pathology with a low prevalence in the general population, but acute complications usually cause sudden death. The etiology is often nonatherosclerotic in the thoracic aorta, but atherosclerotic in the abdominal aorta. Genetic structural malformations cause weakness of the aortic wall resulting in enlargement, whereas bleeding in the atheroma plaques begins aneurysmal vicious circle. The important issue is the implementation of preventive medicine, and one time screening of the body can be helpful for early diagnosis of aortic aneurysms without any sign and symptoms. The rapid growth or significant symptoms are early indications for open or endovascular intervention. In spite of surgical treatment of aortic aneurysms based on open approaches, endovascular repair has gained widespread acceptance due to percutaneous applicability and has been considered the first treatment option in the last years.

Prof. Dr. Kaan Kırali
Head of the Department of Cardiac Transplantation and Ventricular Assist Device
Kartal Koşuyolu YIEA Hospital
Istanbul, Turkey

Department of Cardiovascular Surgery
Faculty of Medicine, Sakarya University
Sakarya, Turkey

Section 1

Introduction

Chapter 1

Introductory Chapter: Limits of Aortic Aneurysm

Kaan Kirali

Additional information is available at the end of the chapter

http://dx.doi.org/10.5772/66679

1. Introduction

The aorta, with its four-dimensional structure, is a complex organ that shows anatomical, functional, embryological, etiological, structural, pathological, dilatational, and spatial variations with limits. Geometrical inequality of the aorta in three-dimensional plane complicates measurement, diagnosis, and therapeutic interventions (open surgery, endovascular, or hybrid procedures) of pathologic segments. Fourth dimensional plane is dependent on cardiac cycles, which change functionally the form and configuration of each segment of the aorta. The requirements of this functional variation of the aorta are maintained by major components: extracellular matrix, elastin, and collagen (predominantly types I and III) [1]. During cardiac systole, the proximal aorta compensates pressure and volume loads (capacitance) and canalizes them distally during diastole through recoil (elastance). The proximal aorta is enrichment of elastic fibers and a relative paucity of collagen (elastin/collagen ratio is 2:1 in thoracal aorta), when compared with more distal aortic segments (collagen/elastin ratio is 2:1 in abdominal aorta). Upper parts of the aorta have more elastic structure to adapt this higher dynamic variation, and elastic fibers show dynamic lengthening and contraction in response to pressure and volume loads, as well as in main branches. This behavior in healthy proximal aorta absorbs and transfers kinetic energy resulted by the left ventricle to transport into the aorta-ejected blood volume toward distally, so that this energy does not cause any pathologic change (dilatation, dissection, outward compression) at the aortic wall. Collagens provide tensile strength and stiffness to the tissue to resist rupture and efficiently propagate pressure waves, especially in distal aorta and in large arteries. This resistance in healthy mid- and distal aorta adsorbs and weakens the kinetic energy carried by blood flow, so that this energy does not result mechanical complications (rupture, bleeding, inward occlusion) at the aortic wall.

The aorta shows different behavior above and below the diaphragm due to different embryologic development of vascular smooth muscular layer. Different segments of the aorta are comprised of cells originating from the neural crest, mesenchyme, and splanchnic mesoderm with a clear difference depending upon the segment. During embryologic development, the thoracic aorta above the ligamentum arteriosum (proximal thoracic aorta) consists by cells from the neural crest commonly with a constant ratio of aortic diameter to medial thickness, whereas the thoracoabdominal aorta below the ligamentum (distal thoracic and abdominal aorta) originates by cells from the mesoderm and the thickness of each unit is expanded during maturation. The media composed of concentric bands of elastin, collagen, and vascular smooth muscle cells provides viscoelasticity; on the other hand, that is the location of degradative remodeling responsible for aneurysm formation. The proximal aorta formed by neural crest is vulnerable against genetic malformation and degradation, which conduct primarily luminal enlargement of the aorta. Proximal aortic dilatation characterizes usually with true aneurysm formation including all aortic wall layers without rupture and clots. The distal aorta formed by mesenchyme is inclined to atherosclerotic changes, which induce first luminal narrowing of the aorta. Distal aortic dilatation characterizes often with pseudoaneurysm formation devoid of all aortic wall layers with rupture and clots.

The etiology of aneurysmal development is often nonatherosclerotic (genetic) in the thoracic aorta, but atherosclerotic in the abdominal aorta [2, 3]. Nonatherosclerotic aneurysm includes inflammation and degeneration. Especially, different aortitis (Takayasu, giant cell arteritis, isolated thoracic arteritis, Behçet disease, syphilis, rheumatic aortitis, etc.) causes granulomatous inflammation with coagulative necrosis and elasticophagia, intimal proliferation, and obliteration without fibrinoid necrosis of the vasa vasorum, and aneurysmal formation if fibrosis is delayed [4]. Genetic disorders cause weakness of the tissues due to loss of structural integrity via specific gene mutations (Marfan syndrome, Loeys-Dietz syndrome, etc.) resulting in cystic medial necrosis, elastic fiber fragmentation, contractile dysfunction, and collagen deposition [5]. Atherosclerotic aneurysm includes atheroma, calcifications, penetrating ulcers, and subadventitial pseudoaneurysms. When atheromatous lesion extends into the media with loss of elastic fibers, the aortic wall is thinned and results in aneurysmal formation. Dissection of blood between intima and media at the ulcer area causes associated psuedoaneurysmal dilatation. Inflammatory aneurysm is characterized by lipids or products of lipid oxidation in the aortic adventitia, extensive adventitial thickening, medial and adventitial fibrosis via lymphoplasmacytic infiltrate, and adhesion to the surrounding retroperitoneal structures.

Aortic aneurysm is a well-known pathology, which can be limited in a segment or spread whole the thoracoabdominal aorta with or without its major branches. Excessive enlargement causes compression symptoms and signs, but its fatal progress is dependent on mechanical complications such as rupture, dissection, fistulization, occlusion, etc. Because aortic aneurysm often has a silent clinical nature until fatal rupture (silent killer), no patient can have time to arrive to hospital when aneurysm is acutely ruptured; however, chronic healing of mechanical complications of aortic aneurysm can give a chance to be diagnosed and treated surgically or endovascularly. The prevalence of aortic aneurysm (>5 cm) is 0.16–0.34% in the general population and the annual incidence of first detected aortic aneurysm (>5 cm) is 5–10 patients/100,000 people (0.005–0.01%), which increases with time and age. At this decade, aortic aneurysm has increased up to 19th leading cause of death (0.64% of the first 20 reasons) in all age groups, but it has reached up to 15th leading pathology of mortality (0.69% of the first 20 reasons) in individuals over 65 years [6]. On the other hand, the true ratio of aortic aneurysm resulting in sudden death must be higher than expected or recorded due to false classification as an acute coronary syndrome (estimated between 2 and 7.5%). That is the fact that aortic aneurysm has an increasing appearance rate in the last decades due to *de novo* cases and/or improvement of imaging modalities. Preventive medicine has a critical role for early diagnosis and reducing of the prevalence in general population. Preventive screening of population with positive family history, profusely predictors, and advanced age provides early diagnosis in asymptomatic patients with an unpredictable, but acceptable devastation of health budgets; whereas periodically screening of diagnosed patients is the gold standard to follow-up patients and to decide initiative time. In spite of excessive improvements in medical technology, health-care policy, interventional therapy techniques, and medical follow-up provide successfully results after aortic aneurysm repair. Sudden death is still the main risk and complication of aortic aneurysms. Avoidance from atherosclerotic risk factors, continuance of physical activity, and maintenance of healthy lifestyle are key points of preventive medical care.

There are two major spatial aneurysm types (**Table 1**). Thoracic aortic aneurysm (TAA) develops in all age groups and is not associated with cardiovascular risk factors, but it can occur as an isolated pathology or it can be associated with different pathologies (**Table 2**) [7]. Most of them are presented syndromic (part of a systemic connective tissue disorder) or nonsyndromic (part of a sporadic structural disorder). The aneurysmal dilatation of the proximal thoracic aorta can be often dependent on a genetic connective tissue disorder with mostly autosomal dominant inheritance or other types, which acts as multisystemic syndrome. The structural malformation of the aortic valve is a common situation, especially bicuspid aortic valve that increases the annular growing speed at least 50% than the normal tricuspid aortic valve. Intracranial aneurysm is the most important concomitant arterial dilatation, which may result in permanent or

1. Thoracic aortic aneurysm
- **a.** Sinus of Valsalva aneurysm
- **b.** Aortic root aneurysm
- **c.** Ascending aorta aneurysm
- **d.** Aortic arch aneurysm
- **e.** Descending aorta aneurysm
- **f.** Combined

2. Abdominal aortic aneurysm
- **a.** Suprarenal
- **b.** Infrarenal
- **c.** Combined
- **d.** Integrated (with iliac arteries)

3. Thoracoabdominal aortic aneurysm
- **a.** Type I (from LSA to CA)
- **b.** Type II (from LSA to IB)
- **c.** Type III (from sixth intercostal space to IB)
- **d.** Type IV (from subdiaphragmatic segment to IB)
- **e.** Type V (from sixth intercostal space to RA)

CA, celiac axis; IB, iliac bifurcation; LSA, left subclavian artery; RA, renal artery.

Table 1. Spatial variations of aortic aneurysms.

1. Intracranial aneurysm (up to 9%)
2. Multisegment involvement of the thoracoabdominal aorta (up to 20–25%)
3. Aortic arch anomalies (up to 20%)

- **a.** Bovine aortic arch (double carotid branching from the brachiocephalic trunk)
- **b.** Isolated left vertebral artery
- **c.** Aberrant right subclavian artery

4. Bicuspid aorta (up to 20–80%)
5. Familial history (up to 20%)
6. Several genetic transition signs (thumb-palm sign)
7. Temporal arteritis
8. Simple renal cyst, polycystic kidney
9. Inguinal hernias

Table 2. Associated pathologies with thoracic aortic aneurysms.

temporary neurologic events, and adversely affect the natural prognosis or surgical outcomes of TAA. Multilevel involvement of the whole aorta is not uncommon and combined aneurysmal enlargement of two different aortic segments worsens fatal risks or surgery. Aortic arch anomalies do not affect the natural course, but they can complicate the pathologic course after complications or surgical repair of TAA. Abdominal aortic aneurysm (AAA) is usually isolated, but it can be associated with TAA in 10–15% of cases. The etiology is different and multifactorial, which cannot affect thoracal aortic segments (**Table 3**) [8]. Smoking and familial history are the main predictors, but also several genetic and inflammatory factors can cause this pathology [9]. Other vascular aneurysms, especially involvement of iliac arteries, are not seldom due to spreading directly or separately [10]. Increased cardiovascular risk factors enforce combined surgical intervention for coronary artery disease [11]. The basic presentation of AAAs is a pseudoaneurysm developed after rupture or perforation of aneurysm sac, which wraps the pathologic segment and supports with attached surrounding tissues against fatal hemorrhage.

Aortic aneurysms grow very slowly during life and overall growth rate is 0.12 cm/year in adults, where it is slower at the ascending aorta (0.1 cm/year) than those at the descending aorta (0.3 cm/year) [12]. As a large elastic artery, definition of aneurysmatic development of the aorta is an enlargement greater than 1.5 times the expected threshold diameter, which are 4 cm for the suprarenal aorta and 3 cm for the infrarenal aorta. The dilatation reaches a hinge diameter in the whole aorta at which the rate of mechanical complications (rupture, dissection) increases exponentially. This borderline diameter is 6 cm for the ascending aorta and 7 cm for the descending aorta. These limits can be used in asymptomatic patients as cut-

1. Smoking
2. Advance age
3. Male
4. Family history
5. Atherosclerosis
6. Hypertension
7. Hypercholesterolemia
8. Other vascular aneurysm

Table 3. Risk factors for abdominal aortic aneurysms.

off value for surgery, but we take down both limits below 6 cm because of 95% of asymptomatic patients have death as a first symptom and we accept the upper limit 5.5 cm in patients without and 5 cm with a risk factor such as Marfan syndrome, bicuspid aortic valve, and family history of sudden death. On the other hand, any symptom caused by aneurysm dilatation (continue retrosternal pain for ascending or interscapular back pain for descending aneurysms) is the cut-off value for surgical treatment regardless of size.

Surgical repair of aortic aneurysms is the definitive treatment procedure with an acceptable hospital mortality and morbidity rates, complication-free long-term survival, and lesser requirement of any reintervention [13–17]. In spite of surgical treatment of aortic aneurysms based on open approaches, endovascular repair has gained widespread acceptance due to percutaneous applicability and is considered the first treatment option in the last years [18]. Open

1. Mortality
2. Stroke
3. Spinal cord injury
4. Renal insufficiency
5. Pulmonary insufficiency

Table 4. Major complications of surgical repair of aortic aneurysms.

conventional surgery remains the standard treatment, but technical complexity increases with more extensive dissection, higher clamp site, prolonged visceral ischemia, and more extensive reconstruction [19]. Major complications are the main drawbacks and hesitations of surgical repair (**Table 4**). To improve intraoperative and early postoperative outcomes, endovascular approaches for aortic aneurysms have evolved and revealed that total endovascular repair with or without hybrid surgical procedures allows reducing operative mortality and morbidity as well as simplifying the intervention and avoiding from complicated steps such as aortic cross-clamping, thoracotomy, single-lung ventilation, and prolonged ischemic time. On the other hand, the presence of several risk factors continues to limit the application of endovascular approaches (**Table 5**). Low- and high-risk patients are not true candidates for hybrid procedure due to high rates of mortality and morbidities and procedural complica-

1. Large aortic seals
2. Short neck (<2 cm)
3. Severe calcified aorta
4. Previously thoracic and/or abdominal surgery
5. Involvement of the visceral arteries
6. Limited life expectancy
7. High-risk patients
a. Unstable angina, malign arrhythmia, recurrent congestive heart failure
b. Left ventricular dysfunction (LVEF < 25%)
c. Vital capacity < 1.8 L
d. Resting pO_2 < 60 mmHg and pCO_2 > 50 mmHg
e. Serum creatinine > 2.5 mg/dL

LVEF, left ventricular ejection fraction; pO_2, oxygen partial pressure; pCO_2, partial pressure of carbon dioxide.

Table 5. Factors complicating endovascular interventions.

tions, but this approach is useful in patients who require creation of definitive landing zone [20]. Another frequent choice of endovascular repair is ruptured AAAs due to easier and more noninvasive nature of the procedure, whereas open surgical treatment has similar or better outcomes [21].

Author details

Kaan Kirali

Address all correspondence to: imkbkirali@yahoo.com

1 Department of Cardiovascular Surgery, Kartal Kosuyolu YIEA Hospital, Istanbul, Turkey

2 Department of Cardiovascular Surgery, Faculty of Medicine, Sakarya University, Sakarya, Turkey

References

[1] Lindsay ME, Dietz HC. The genetic basis of aortic aneurysm. Cold Spring Harb Perspect Med 2014;4(9):a015909.

[2] Ruddy JM, Jones JA, Ikonomidis JS. Pathophysiology of thoracic aortic aneurysm (TAA): Is it not one uniform aorta? Role of embryologic origin. Prog Cardiovasc Dis 2013;56(1):68–73.

[3] Lu H, Rateri DL, Bruemmer D, Cassis LA, Daugherty A. Novel mechanisms of abdominal aortic aneurysms. Curr Atheroscler Rep 2012;14(5):402–412.

[4] Ikeda Y. Aortic aneurysm: Etiopathogenesis and clinicopathologic correlations. Ann Vasc Dis 2016;9(2):73–79.

[5] Lindsay ME, Dietz HC. Lessons on the pathogenesis of aneurysm from heritable conditions. Nature 2011; 473(7347):308–316.

[6] WISQARS leading causes of death reports, 1999–2007. 2015. Available online: http://webappa.cdc.gov/sasweb/ncipc/leadcaus10.html (Accessed 15.11.15).

[7] Ziganshin BA, Elefteriades JA. Guilt by association: A paradigm for detection of silent aortic disease. Ann Cardiothorac Surg 2016;5(3):174–187.

[8] Kuivaniemi H, Ryer EJ, Elmore JR, Tromp G. Understanding the pathogenesis of abdominal aortic aneurysms. Expert Rev Cardiovasc Ther 2015;13(9):975–987.

[9] Erentuğ V, Bozbuğa N, Ömeroğlu SN, Ardal H, Eren E, Elevli MG, Güzelmeriç F, Kirali K, Akinci E, Yakut C. Rupture of abdominal aortic aneurysms in Behçet's disease. Ann Vasc Surg 2003;17(6):682–685.

[10] Robinson D, Mees B, Verhagen H, Cheun J. Aortic aneurysms: Screening, surveillance and referral. Australian Family Phys 2013;42(6):364–369.

[11] Gürbüz A, Kirali K, Tuncer A, Şişmanoğlu M, Yakut C. Combined transdiaphragmatic MIDCAB with right gastroepiploic artery and abdominal aortic aneurysm repair. Cardiovasc Surg 2000;8(6):503–506.

[12] 1Elefteriades JA, Farkas EA. Thoracic aortic aneurysm: Clinically pertinent controversies and uncertainties. J Am Coll Cardiol 2010;55(9):841–857.

[13] Sarikaya S, Adademir T, Elibol A, Büyükbayrak F, Onk A, Kirali K. Surgery for ruptured sinus of Valsalva aneurysm: 25-year experience with 55 patients. Eur J Cardiothorac Surg 2013;43(3):591–596.

[14] Mataraci I, Polat A, Kiran B, Caliskan A, Tuncer A, Erentug V, Kirali K, Isik O, Yakut C. Long-term results of aortic root replacement: 15 years' experience. Ann Thorac Surg 2009;87(6):1783–1788.

[15] Mataraci I, Kirali K, Ökten M, Aksüt M, Erentuğ V, Balkanay M, Akinci E, Yakut C. Surgical repair of thoracoabdominal aortic aneurysms and dissections using the femoro-femoral distal perfusion technique Turk Gogus Kalp Dama 2009;17(1):1–7.

[16] Kirali K. Surgical strategy in aortic aneuyrsms: Modified Bentall – aortic valve sparing surgery. Turkiye Klinikleri J Cardiovasc Surg-Special Topics 2012;4(1):7–17.

[17] Özen Y, Sarikaya S, Rabuş MB, Aydin E, Dedemoğlu M, Kirali K. A comparison of hiatal and thoracic clamping in ruptured abdominal aort aneurysms. Türk Gogus Kalp Dama 2015;23(2):280–284.

[18] Oderich GS, Mendes BC, Gloviczki P, Kalra M, Duncan AA, Bower TC. Current role and future directions of hybrid repair of thoracoabdominal aortic aneurysms. Perspect Vasc Surg Endovasc Ther 2012;24(1):14–22.

[19] Kirali K, Göksedef D, Kayalar N. Surgical treatment in intrathoracic aortic aneurysms. In: Duran E (ed). Cardiovascular Surgery. First Edition. Istanbul, Turkey: Çapa Medicine Pub; 2004:1587–1631.

[20] Orr N, Minion D, Bobadilla JL. Thoracoabdominal aortic aneurysm repair: Current endovascular perspectives. Vasc Health Risk Manag 2014;10:493–505.

[21] Patelis N, Moris D, Karaolanis G, Georgopoulos S. Endovascular vs. open repair for ruptured abdominal aortic aneurysm. Med Sci Monit Basic Res 2016;22:34–44.

Section 2

Proximal Aortic Aneurysm

Chapter 2

Isolated Aortic Root Aneurysms

Kaan Kırali and Deniz Günay

Additional information is available at the end of the chapter

http://dx.doi.org/10.5772/66963

Abstract

The aortic root has a complex anatomy due to a combination of several anatomical structures based on simple and consistent work in it. It is a hollow cylinder with three bulges, which have the main functional effect on the aortic valve opening-closing cycle and coronary circulation. Aneurysm is defined as a dilation of a blood vessel segment having ≥50% increase in diameter, whereas annuloaortic ectasia represents a diffuse dilation <50% of the normal diameter of the related vessel segment. Aortic root aneurysms mostly occur by degenerative processes as compared with primarily atherosclerotic changes in the descending and abdominal aortas: medial fragmentation, smooth muscle cells necrosis, and elastic fiber fragmentations with cystic spaces in the media filled with mucoid material. Because of the elevated mortality risk associated with complications, an effective aortic root aneurysm management depends on reduction the risk of death, rupture, and dissection. Conventional open heart surgery is the essential procedure for isolated aortic root replacement and a type of procedure (valve replacement or sparing) could be selected due to the pathology. An extensive aortic root replacement technique is the only option to rebuild the left ventricular outflow tract due to the reconstruction of the neo aortoventricular continuity in the aortic root abscess.

Keywords: aortic root, root aneurysm, annuloaortic ectasia, aortic root replacement, aortic valve sparing, Bentall, Flanged, Cabrol, remodeling, reimplantation, extensive root replacement

1. Introduction

The aortic root is the first anatomical part of the aorta and also a functional bridge between the left ventricular outflow tract and ascending aorta, which lies between the ventriculoaortic junction (VAJ) and sinotubular junction (STJ). The aortic root has a complex anatomy due to a combination of several anatomical structures based on simple and consistent work in it. This complex combination provides several unique functional futures. On the other hand, several pathological processes disrupting this anatomo-physiological structure lead to functional, morphological, and hemodynamic disturbances. Detailed understanding of the complex anatomy of the aortic root leads to the development of many sophisticated, but functional and artistic surgical techniques. This chapter focuses only on the abnormal enlargement of the aortic root caused by different pathologies, complicated or not, and surgical treatment options.

2. Definition

Generally, two terms are used to describe the aortic root enlargement: aneurysm and annuloaortic ectasia. Aneurysm is defined as a dilation of a blood vessel segment having ≥50% increase in diameter compared with the expected normal diameter. True aneurysm involves all three layers of the arterial wall, but a pseudoaneurysm does not involve any anatomical layer of the aortic wall and is surrounded by thrombosis and/or surrounding tissues. Annuloaortic ectasia represents a diffuse dilation <50% of the normal diameter of the related vessel segment. The aortic root does not have a tubular or cylindrical shape with the same diameter at all levels; on the contrary, it has variable diameters at different levels. Normal dimensions of the aortic root are different between genders and they also varies depending on age and body surface area (BSA): annulus diameter is approximately 26 ± 3 and 23 ± 2 mm, sinus Valsalva diameter is 34 ± 3 and 30 ± 3 mm, and STJ diameter 29 ± 3 and 27 ± 4 mm in male and female population, respectively [1]. Calculated normal aortic diameter indexes (diameter/BSA) can be useful during surgical treatment to choice a patient-appropriate tubular graft, especially to prevent any patient-prosthesis mismatch: annular diameter index is approximately 13 ± 1 mm/m^2, sinus Valsalva diameter index 19 ± 1 mm/m^2, and STJ diameter index 15 ± 1 mm/m^2 [2].

3. Functional anatomy

The aortic root has a truncated corn shape with the semilunar attachments of the leaflets, sinuses, interleaflet triangles, and commissures (**Figure 1**). The top of the aortic root is created by the distal circumferential plane joining the crests of three commissures and named as the STJ. The bulged mid-portion of the aortic root has three sinuses of Valsalva and it is like a three-leaflet clover in two-dimensional view (**Figure 2**): left coronary sinus (LCS), right coronary sinus (RCS), and noncoronary sinus (NCS). The base of the aortic root is shaped as a zone between the left ventricle and aorta because there is not a true single-circular annular attachment of three aortic leaflets. This anatomic VAJ is a circular zone between lower and upper rings: *The basal ring* or anatomic aortic annulus is the circular ring at the nadirs of three sinuses of Valsalva which is supported by the left ventricular muscle beneath the RCS and ½ anterior LCS, and by the fibrous aortic-mitral curtain beneath the NCS and ½ posterior LCS. This level is the narrowest circular level of the aortic valve. *The ventriculo-arterial ring* or the hemodynamic aortic annulus is the circular ring at the top of the muscular structure of the sinuses of Valsalva, which is supported only by the aortic wall. The interleaflet triangles

http://dx.doi.org/10.5772/66963

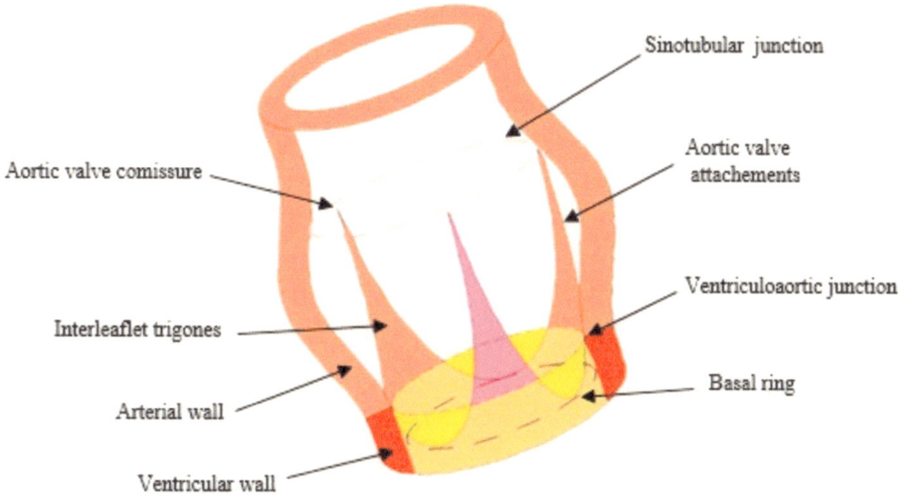

Figure 1. Aortic root.

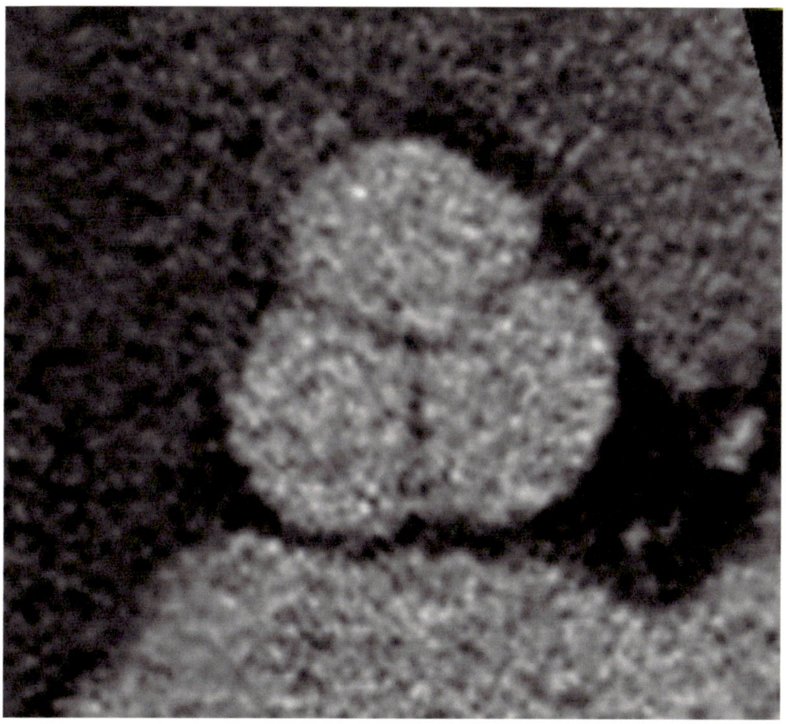

Figure 2. Two-dimensional computed tomographic view of three sinuses of Valsalva like a three-leaflet clover.

have special features because of their anatomical neighborhood relationships. The right interleaflet triangle separates RCS and NCS, it has continuity with the membranous septum and both built the right fibrous trigone. The most important anatomic structure in this area is His bundles, which lie just below the triangle. The posterior interleaflet triangle separates NCS and LCS, it has continuity with aortico-mitral valvular curtain and both built the left fibrous trigone, where guides to posterior aortic root enlargement techniques. The left interleaflet triangle has muscular structure and separates LCS and RCS, which is the closest part of the aortic root to the pulmonary trunk.

The aortic root is a hollow cylinder with three bulges, which have the main functional effect on the aortic valve opening-closing cycle and coronary circulation. In fact, the aortic root has two-sided asymmetrical structure [3]. *The first asymmetry* is in the longitudinal axis, and the mean heights of each sinus of Valsalva (NCS > RCS > LCS) and each interleaflet triangle (posterior ≥ right > left) are not same, and the free margin lengths of the leaflets correspond this asymmetry [4]. This asymmetry shapes the aortic root as a conic cuff, whereas the NCS is slightly larger, and this pattern determines an angle of upper tilt (from the posterior interleaflet triangle to the NCS) between the plane at the VAJ and STJ with a mean value of 11° [5]. *The second asymmetry* is in the circumferential axis and the diameters of the aortic root are different (sinus of Valsalva > VAJ > STJ ≈ 1.34 > 1.1 > 1). The diameter of the STJ is 10–12% smaller than those of the VAJ; however, the upper parts of the commissures attach just below the STJ and make a virtual ring with the same diameter of the VAJ.

The aortic root changes its overall configuration from a cone to a cylinder and from a cylinder to an inverted cone according to left ventricular filling and contraction [6]. Because the aortic leaflets attach in the shape of a three-pointed crown spanning the entire vertical extent of the aortic root from the VAJ to the STJ, it is more meaningful to discuss "the aortic valve apparatus" (**Table 1**). This functional apparatus organizes ventricular and arterial hemodynamics, and it works with an elegant mechanism. Every part of this apparatus has own function during the cardiac cycle. The aortic valve passively opens and closes in response to pressure differences between the left ventricle and aorta. The expansion of the VAJ at the preejectional phase before aortic valve opening helps to decrease the coaptation area among the leaflets

1.	Ascending aorta
2.	Sinotubular ring (junction)
3.	Sinuses of Valsalva
4.	Commissures
5.	Interleaflet triangles
6.	Aortic leaflets
7.	Ventriculoaortic ring (junction)
8.	Left ventricle

Table 1. Aortic valve apparatus.

http://dx.doi.org/10.5772/66963

and to separate the leaflets under minimal stresses (20% of total opening), and the aortic valve opening is completed rapidly by the ejection phase. The STJ expands approximately 12% during systole and the aortic root gets more cylindrical shape in the longitudinal axis, where inflow and outflow effective orifice areas of the aortic root become similar, and this configuration allows a zero resistance to flow throughout the aortic root during every ejection. Sinuses of Valsalva have the main effect on the coronary blood circulation, whereas they permit aortic valve opening during systole without blocking of the coronary artery ostia and simplify aortic valve closing at the end of systole without any tension.

The aortic root with this complex structure maintains the functional capacity of the aortic valve and the conversion of intermittent and irregular high blood volume from the left ventricle to regular and laminar blood flow even in variable hemodynamic conditions. Both the STJ and VAJ provide aortic valve coaptation, but the outflow part of the aortic root is the main structure that promotes aortic valve coaptation, whereas it hangs all three commissures during the diastole. Any significant dilatation of these rings can cause aortic regurgitation, whereas enlargement of the STJ more than 110% of the VAJ diameter results severe aortic insufficiency.

4. Histology and pathohistology

The aortic leaflets are covered by a continuous layer of endothelial cells with a smooth surface on the ventricular side and numerous ridges on the arterial side. The aortic leaflets are attached to the sinus wall via a very dense collagenous meshwork hinged to the annulus, so they transmit the stress on the leaflets to the aortic wall during diastole. The right and posterior interleaflet triangles consist of a thinned fibrous wall of the aorta, whereas the left interleaflet triangle is supported by muscular tissue and only fibrous at its apex. Interleaflet triangles contain primary collagen fibers; in contrast, sinuses of Valsalva contain concentric elastic lamella.

The aortic wall has three layers: tunica intima, tunica media, and tunica externa (adventitia), which are separated from each other with a thin membrane: membrana elastica interna (between intima and media) and membrana elastica externa (between media and adventitia). The intima is composed of single layers of endothelial cells arranged in the direction of the vessel. The subendothelial connective tissue is arranged in the same manner as the endothelial cells. The media is composed of circular arranged structures: smooth muscle cells, elastic fibers, collagen, and proteoglycans. The adventitia is arranged in a longitudinal fashion and composed of collagen fibers of type I. Although the wall of the sinuses is principally arranged in this manner, the thickness of its wall is significantly thinner compared with the ascending aorta and STJ [7].

The tunica media of the aortic root comprises concentric layers around the lumen, which consist two elastic lamellae and intervening tissue between them. The elastic lamellae include collagen fibers (type I-III-V) and fibronectin, and they are interconnected by a network of elastic and collagen fibers, and proteoglycans. Smooth muscle cells are also in contact with fibrillin-1 and type VI collagen containing bundles of microfibrils (oxytalan fibers), and they have a basal lamina-like layer connecting them to each other and oxytalan fibers [8]. There are many types of proteoglycans in vascular walls such as collagen-associated dermatan sulfate proteoglycan, cell-associated heparin sulfate proteoglycan, and interstitial chondroitin sulfate proteoglycan. The constituents of the arterial wall are responsible for mechanical properties, and the ability of the arterial vessel is essential to prevent or limit any permanent deformation. Elastic fibers providing the elasticity and compliance of the arterial wall comprise elastin and microfibrils such as fibulins, fibrillins, and microfibril-associated glycoproteins.

Aortic root aneurysms mostly occur by degenerative processes as compared with primarily atherosclerotic changes in the descending and abdominal aortas. The elastin content of the aorta decreases distally and in the abdominal aorta it is less than half of that in the ascending aorta. Degenerative processes mean medial fragmentation, smooth muscle cells necrosis, and elastic fiber fragmentations with cystic spaces in the media filled with mucoid material. There is a disorganization and breakdown of the elastin network and its interconnections with the collagen network and other components of the aortic wall. The collagen structure also alters specifically and significantly: collagens type I and III decrease, while collagens alpha-1 (XI) and V increase [9]. Smooth muscle cell impairment and increased amounts of the vacuolated basophilic material are prominent.

Matrix metalloproteinases play an important role in connective tissue homeostasis, and in fragmentation of extracellular matrix elements via digestion of elastin and collagen fibers [10, 11]. Disharmony of matrix metalloproteinases activity causes connective tissue impairment. Blockade of plasmin formation by overexpression of plasminogen activator inhibitor-1 prevents the formation of aneurysms by inhibiting metalloproteinase activation. And also, local overexpression of the tissue inhibitor of matrix metalloproteinases can prevent aneurysmal degeneration and rupture. Inflammation characterized with leukocyte and lymphocyte infiltration is greater in the aneurysmal aortic wall compared to nonaneurysmal aortas, especially in some inflammatory disorders. Many inflammatory mediators (interferon-γ, interleukin-1 β, TNF-α, IL-6, TGF-β) increase in degenerative aortic aneurysms and their disharmony stimulates aneurysm formation [12, 13]. Genetic abnormalities can also cause this disharmony that results abnormal functions and structures in aortic wall. These disorganizations can cause early degeneration of the vascular wall and aneurysmal formation. Some genetic defects or mutations causing specific diseases are well described: *gene ACTA2* to familial thoracic aortic aneurysm; *gene TGFBR1* to Loeys-Dietz syndrome; *gene TGFBR2* to familial thoracic aortic aneurysm, Marfan syndrome, and Loeys-Dietz syndrome; *gene FBN1* to Marfan syndrome; *gene* COL3A1 to Ehlers-Danlos syndrome.

5. Pathophysiology

Aortic root aneurysm occurs due to decreased connective tissue strength or elevated pressure in the aorta. High content of an elastic fiber in the medial layer of the aortic root provides

http://dx.doi.org/10.5772/66963

expansion during systole acting as a reservoir and stores kinetic energy resulting by left ventricular contraction as potential energy in the aortic wall. In diastole, elastic recoil returns the aortic root to its original form back and transforms the stored potential energy back to kinetic energy to start aortic wave motion for forward blood flow. Several pathological changes lead to degenerative processes in the elastic media and decreasing the strength of the aortic wall connective tissue.

The coupling between mechanical stress and the biochemical changes leading an aneurysmal formation is not well elucidated. Several adversely changed mechanisms such as decreased aortic wall compliance, broken cross-sectional symmetry, and disrupted stress-strain relationships increase intraluminal systolic impulse stress and aortic wall tension, which active predate dilatation formation (tension = pressure × radius). Because the inner curvature of the aortic root is adherent to the pulmonary artery, the NCS is the most affected part of the root and the typical enlargement occurs at the STJ level, especially in aortic root dilatation associated with ascending aortic aneurysm. Synchronously involvement of three sinuses causes a symmetrical aneurysmal dilatation (resembling a pear).

6. Etiology

There are different specific etiologies causing aortic root aneurysm (**Table 2**). Most of them have genetic origin, but the most common etiology is *bicuspid aortopathy*. The prevalence of aortic dilation ranges from 20 to 84% in bicuspid aortic valve (BAV) disease [14]. In patients with BAV disease, three enlargement patterns are described according to whether the maximal aortic diameter is at the level of the sinuses of Valsalva, the STJ, or the ascending aorta. Four subtypes of BAV disease are identified with different forms of aortic dilation: aortic root alone (13%), ascending aorta alone (10%), ascending aorta and proximal transverse arch (28%), and from the aortic root to the proximal transverse arch (45%) [15]. There is a relationship between the morphology of the ascending aorta and the valve fusion pattern: left coronary cusp-right coronary cusp type associated with ascending aorta and aortic root dilation; right coronary cusp-noncoronary cusp type associated with only ascending aorta dilatation. Isolated *sinuses of Valsalva aneurysm* develop because of either a congenital defect or acquired pathologies such as endocarditis, aortic dissection, or iatrogenic causes [16]. The most common cause is weakness between the media and the annulus fibrosus of the aorta, which can cause aneurysmal enlargement. The RCS is most frequently affected, followed by the NCS. The aneurysm can rupture into any of low-pressure cardiac chambers, especially into the right-sided ones, to form an aortico-cardiac fistula. Aortic valve abnormalities and incompetence occur especially after rupture. Genetic diseases with autosomal dominant penetrance usually involve multiple organ systems, and their common involvement is the aorta. The most common genetic disease with an aortic root aneurysm is the **Marfan's syndrome**, which is associated with mutations in the FBN-1 gene and has autosomal dominant heredity [17]. Approximately 3/4 of patients with Marfan's syndrome have aortic root dilatation with or without aortic valve regurgitation and ½ mitral regurgitation.

1. Bicuspid aortic valve disease
2. Sinus of Valsalva aneurysm
3. Genetic diseases
a. Marfan's syndrome
b. Ehlers-Danlos syndrome
c. Loeys-Dietz syndrome
d. Turner syndrome
e. Aneurysm-osteoarthritis syndrome
f. Nonsyndromic familial thoracic aortic aneurysms
4. Familial aneurysms
5. Infection
6. Inflammatory diseases
a. Takayasu's arteritis
b. Giant cell arteritis
c. Behçet's disease
d. Ankylosing spondylitis
e. Wegener's granulomatosis
f. Rheumatoid arthritis

Table 2. Etiology for aortic root aneurysm.

7. Diagnosis

Although clinical symptoms (retrosternal pain, hoarseness, breathless, etc.), examination (aortic valve murmur), and several laboratory testing play a minor role in the diagnosis of the aortic root aneurysms, noninvasive imaging techniques have a major role yielding a view of the total intrathoracic aorta [18]. In the daily practice, transthoracic echocardiography associated with transoesophageal echocardiography is the most frequently used technique for the diagnosis, which should be completed with thoracic computed tomography and/or magnetic resonance imaging, as well as ultrasonography and/or computed tomography for the abdominal aorta. It is recommended to measure diameters at anatomical landmarks perpendicular to the longitudinal axis (antegrade flow in the aortic root and ascending aorta) and to use the same imaging modality with a similar method of measurement in the case of repetitive imaging of the aorta. The aortic annulus should be measured at midsystole from the inner-edge-to-inner edge and all other aortic root measurements (i.e., maximal diameter of the sinuses of Valsalva, the sinotubular junction, and the proximal ascending aorta) should be made at end-diastole. Measurements of maximal diameters of the aortic root should be compared with age- and BSA-related nomograms or to values calculated from specific allometric equations (**Table 3**).

http://dx.doi.org/10.5772/66963

Aortic root	Absolute values (cm)		Indexed values (cm/m^2)	
	Men	Women	Men	Women
Annulus	2.6 ± 0.3	2.3 ± 0.2	1.3 ± 0.1	1.3 ± 0.1
Sinuses of Valsalva	3.4 ± 0.3	3.0 ± 0.3	1.7 ± 0.2	1.8 ± 0.2
Sinotubular junction	2.9 ± 0.3	2.6 ± 0.3	1.5 ± 0.2	1.5 ± 0.2
Proximal ascending aorta	3.0 ± 0.4	2.7 ± 0.4	1.5 ± 0.2	1.6 ± 0.3

Table 3. Aortic root dimensions in normal adults.

Aneurysm surveillance in asymptomatic patients includes ongoing clinical evaluation, the development of symptoms, signs of aneurysm complications, and serial imaging to evaluate the diameter and structure of the aneurysm. Ideally, the serial studies should be performed using the same technique (echocardiography, computed tomographic angiography or magnetic resonance angiography) in the same center for consistency with future comparisons. Aortic valve function and morphology should be evaluated during follow-up; therefore, echocardiographic assessment should be considered in aortic root aneurysm. The surveillance program may be modified based upon the etiology, site, and diameter of the aneurysm at presentation. In general, imaging at 6 months after the initial diagnosis could ensure the stability of the aneurysm and expansion rate. The thoracic aorta expands slowly with the age at a rate of 0.7 mm in women and 0.9 mm in men per decade of life. The expansion rate of the aortic aneurysms is much higher than these values, and a larger diameter of aortic root aneurysms could expands more rapidly than smaller ones like other segments of the aorta: the rate of expansion for large aneurysms (>5 cm) was about 8 mm per year while 2 mm per year for smaller aneurysms (<5 cm).

8. Indications

Once the aortic root aneurysm detected patient should be examined for concomitant diseases, genetically mediated disorders and risk factors. Major life threatening complications are dissection, rupture, and aortic valve regurgitation. Because of the elevated mortality risk associated with complications, an effective aortic root aneurysm management depends on reduction the risk of death, rupture, and dissection. The most important determinant is the diameter of the aneurysm. Other factors, such as a rapidly expanding aortic diameter, concomitant bicuspid aortic valve, or connective tissue disease also increase the risk of rupture.

Medical treatment depends on reducing aortic wall stress and slow down medial degeneration. Lifestyle modifications contain smoking cessation, avoiding intensive exercise, and patient education. Aggressive antihypertensive therapy is the mainstay of pharmacologic management to prevent increased wall stress. If tolerated, a goal of the therapy is

A. Presence of elastopathy
   1. Without risk factors
      a. ≥50 mm
      b. Diameter increase > 3 mm/year
   2. With family history of aortic dissection and/or aortic diameter increase
      a. ≥45 mm
      b. Diameter increase > 3 mm/year

B. Presence of BAV
   1. ≥55 mm
   2. ≥50 mm associated with
      a. Diameter increase > 3 mm/year
      b. Family history of dissection
      c. Coarctation of the aorta
      d. Systemic hypertension
      e. Moderate AI and/or AS
   3. >45 mm when AVR is scheduled

C. Presence of significant aortic valve insufficiency and/or stenosis
   1. ≥50 mm
   2. Diameter increase > 3 mm/year

D. Absence of elastopathy or any risk factor
   1. ≥55 mm
   2. Diameter increase > 5 mm/year

Note: AI = aortic insufficiency; AS = aortic stenosis; AVR = aortic valve replacement; BAV = bicuspid aortic valve.

Table 4. Surgical indications for asymptomatic aortic root aneurysms without dissection.

maintaining a systolic pressure below 120 mmHg. Beta-blockers reduce the contractility of the heart, decrease shear stress, and the impact force of ejected blood on the aorta. Although these beneficial effects, it should be noted that the β-blocker therapy will block the compensatory tachycardia and could precipitate clinical deterioration in aortic regurgitation. Reduction in heart rate is also associated with an even higher stroke volume, which contributes to the elevated systolic pressure in patients with chronic severe aortic regurgitation. On the other hand, patients treated with β-blockers have a significantly lower growth rate (1.2 mm/year) than those without β-blocker treatment (4.2 mm/year), which shows the beneficial effect and the importance of β-blocker medical therapy on aneurysm stabilization [19].

http://dx.doi.org/10.5772/66963

Surgical indication is dependent on the presence of symptoms and diameter measurements of several parts of the ascending aorta. In general, surgical repair of asymptomatic aortic root aneurysm is not recommended until the risk of dissection, rupture or other complications exceeds the risks associated with surgery (**Table 4**). In general, asymptomatic aortic root aneurysms without dissection must be directed to surgical treatment depending upon an aortic diameter (≥5 cm) and speedy expansion rate (≥5 mm/year); however, in the presence of underlying special contributing etiologies these limits should be decreased (≥4.5 cm or ≥3 mm/year or the presence of acute or chronic aortic dissection). Aneurysms can cause symptoms especially in larger diameters. Symptoms could be pioneers of fatal complications, therefore surgery should be considered for symptomatic patients either at smaller diameters of aneurysm.

9. Surgery

Aortic valve replacement (AVR) with supracoronary ascending aorta replacement is the first aortic root surgery operation. The Bentall technique is the first true total aortic root replacement (ARR) procedure, which contains en bloc replacement of the ascending aorta. The modified Bentall technique eliminates wrapping of the native aortic wall over the tubular graft. The Button technique eliminates most of problems regarding to coronary ostial anastomoses via end-to-side reimplantation of the coronary ostia. A interposition graft between the coronary ostia and the composite graft to prevent coronary malposition is especially useful when mobilization of the coronary buttons is often difficult or impossible. Other modifications include leaving a small part of the tubular graft below the prosthetic valve to simplify and secure aortic annular anastomosis [20–22], To simplify proximal annular anastomosis, a prefabricated composite graft with sinus of Valsalva can be chosen [23].

Conventional open heart surgery is the essential procedure for isolated ARR. Urgent surgery is usually preferred for life-threating pathologies of the aortic root, and standard approaches should initially be used for emergent situations or with concomitant cardiac procedures. Some more recent approaches toward more noninvasive surgery can be considered in elective, noncomplicated-isolated aortic root surgery. General anesthesia with full median sternotomy is the standard approach for aortic root surgery, and transesophageal echocardiography is mandatory in cases of aortic valve-sparing procedures. Awake cardiac surgery offers several advantages over general anesthesia, including the absence of tracheal intubation, reduced stress response, lower postoperative arrhythmias, and improved pulmonary outcome [24–26]. This approach may be more beneficial and safer in patients with chronic obstructive pulmonary disease who are frequently rejected for cardiac surgery [27, 28]. This approach should be only used in elective cases with noncomplicated aortic root surgery, whereas general anesthesia remains the preferred option in aortic valve-sparing procedures or in emergency situations. Full median sternotomy is the versatile and most reliable option to reach all sites of the heart, but minimal invasive incisions may be preferred in order to reduce invasivity and adverse effects of full median sternotomy. The full median sternotomy can be restricted only to perform aortic root surgery in the presence of other concomitant cardiac pathologies, otherwise limited median sternotomy techniques are the best approach for isolated aortic root surgery due to shorter hospitalization periods, improved lung functions, reduced trauma effects, and early mobilization. There are two most preferred minimal invasive incision techniques for access into the mediastinum: *J sternotomy* is the most preferred ministernotomy incision in isolated AVR operations [29, 30], but only *upper reverse-T ministernotomy* is an appropriate approach to reach the aortic root and to perform all varieties of aortic root surgeries [31, 32]. After the usual preparations, standard central arterial cannulation is established through the distal ascending aorta or the lateral wall of the mid aortic arch. If any dissection is present at the ascending aorta, the arterial cannulation should be performed through a patent peripheral artery [33]. Venous cannulation is prepared using a thinner single two-staged venous cannula through the right atrial appendage or an appropriate venous cannula through the femoral vein, and venous return is maintained via a negative vacuum venous drainage system. A negative vacuum system is very effective in emptying the heart and can achieve left heart decompression without the use of a vent cannula. A vent cannula is passed through the right upper pulmonary vein into the left atrium. Cardiopulmonary bypass is established at 32°C, but if an extended operation time is predicted, perfusate temperature decreases to 28°C. After cardioplegic arrest is accomplished, myocardial protection is achieved via an antegrade (direct coronary ostia) or a retrograde (through the coronary sinus) route.

Conventional open heart surgery is the essential procedure for isolated ARR and a type of procedure could be selected due to the pathology (**Table 5**). It is always a good idea to keep in mind that the ARR surgery is a life-saving procedure and there are not many drawbacks to the conventional procedures. On the other hand, less invasive or aggressive interventions may be chosen in elective and selective cases [34]. The first goal during ARR is to spare the competent aortic valve if possible. If not possible, the use of a composite graft to replace whole ascending aorta seems the most preferred option during ARR. The first choice of a prosthetic valve for ARR is a mechanical valve due to its simple handling, easy sizing, lower profile, long-term durability, and resistance to mechanical stress. Composite grafts with stentless bioprosthetic valves can be chosen in older patients to avoid valve-related late reoperations. But, using mechanical valve conduits could be changed to the use of bioprosthetic composite grafts in all age groups if the transcatheter methods offer similar or better results when compared to reoperative ARR procedures. Although allografts can be the best option for the total ARR, their availability is very limited in most countries.

9.1. Total aortic root replacement procedures with aortic valve replacement

The modified Bentall technique with mechanical or stentless biological valve is the gold standard for the total ARR (**Figure 3**). The "modified" procedure describes the discontinuation of the practice of wrapping the aortic wall over the graft and the button anastomosis of the

http://dx.doi.org/10.5772/66963

A. Total aortic root replacement
   I. With aortic valve replacement
      1. Modified Bentall procedure
      2. Cabrol procedure
      3. Flanged procedure
      4. Biologic Bentall procedure
         a. Allograft
         b. Xenograft
      5. Ross procedure
   II. Without aortic valve replacement (valve-sparing aortic root replacement)
      1. Remodeling (Yacoub procedure)
      2. Reimplantation (David V procedure)
B. Subtotal aortic root replacement (without aortic valve)
      1. One sinus replacement
      2. Double sinus replacement
      3. Sinus of Valsalva aneurysm repair
C. Extensive aortic root replacement (with aortoventricular base)

Table 5. Aortic root replacement techniques.

coronary ostia rather than as required in the originally described technique. After aortic cross-clamping, a 2 cm transverse aortotomy is performed just above the STJ to visualize the aortic root and leaflets, and then the ascending aorta is divided completely. The second step is resection of aortic sinuses and leaflets, which remains 3–5 mm over from the transected tissues. Preparing the coronary buttons with a 1.5 cm diameter cuff of the aortic wall and mobilizing over a short length to facilitate reimplantation is the last step before composite graft implantation. All other necessary concomitant procedures such as distal anastomosis of coronary bypass grafts and/or valvular repair/replacement are performed before the ARR. To prevent postoperative bleeding from the proximal anastomosis, a reinforcement suture joining the incised edge of the aortic wall and the prosthetic sewing ring can be used [35]. The miniskirt technique has been developed to secure proximal bleeding, where first all interrupted mattress sutures enter the aortic annulus, the sewing ring of the prosthesis and the vascular graft leaving a short segment, and then proximal hemostasis is secured with a running suture by buttressing the aortic remnants and graft edge [20]. Alternatively, a short skirt of Dacron tube can be added to the proximal end of a standard composite graft and sewn to the remaining native aortic wall to wrap the proximal annular anastomosis after the completion of the implantation of this modified composite graft on the aortic annulus [36].

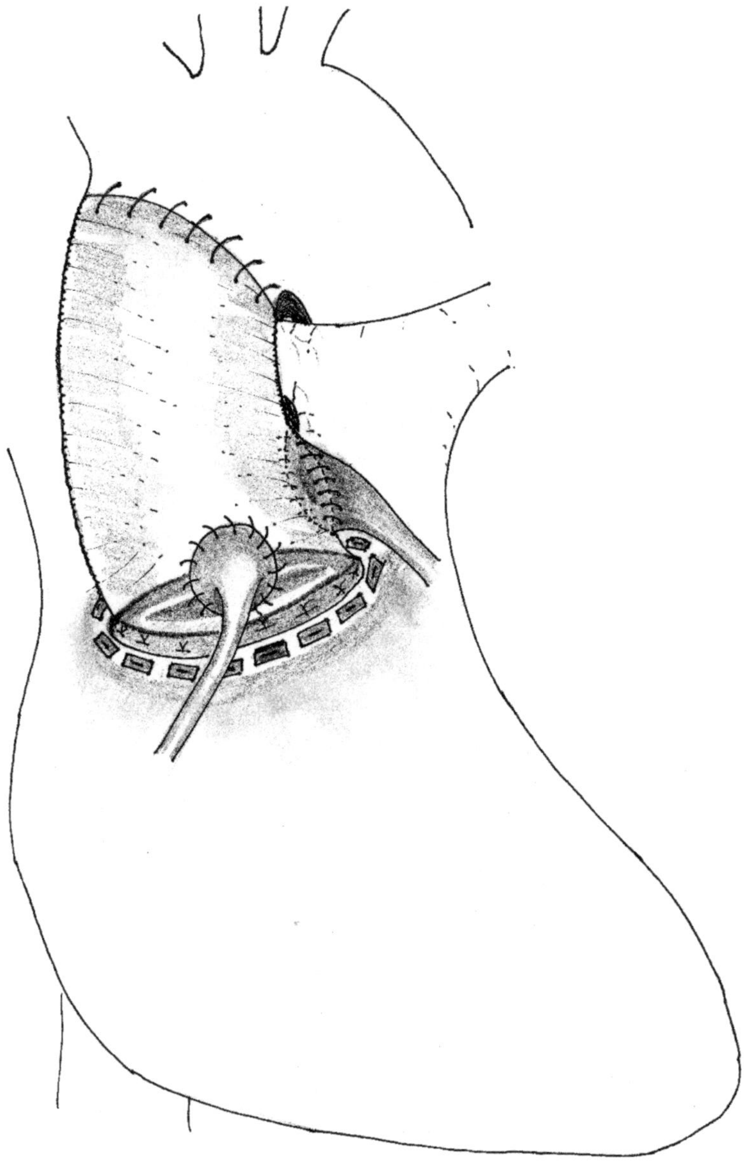

Figure 3. Modified Bentall procedure.

The Cabrol technique is carried out using a "moustache-shaped" interposition tubular graft (8 mm) between coronary ostia and aortic graft (**Figure 4**). This technique can be very useful in reoperation procedures, where the mobilization of the coronary buttons is difficult, and also in severely calcified coronary ostia. Except coronary ostium anastomoses, all operative steps are similar to the modified Bentall procedure, as described in detail above. In some cases with an extremely large aortic diameter at the level of sinuses, the right coronary button anastomosis can be challenging if the mobilization of the right coronary button is not adequate to reach the relatively small prosthetic neoaorta. Because this technique has worse outcomes

http://dx.doi.org/10.5772/66963

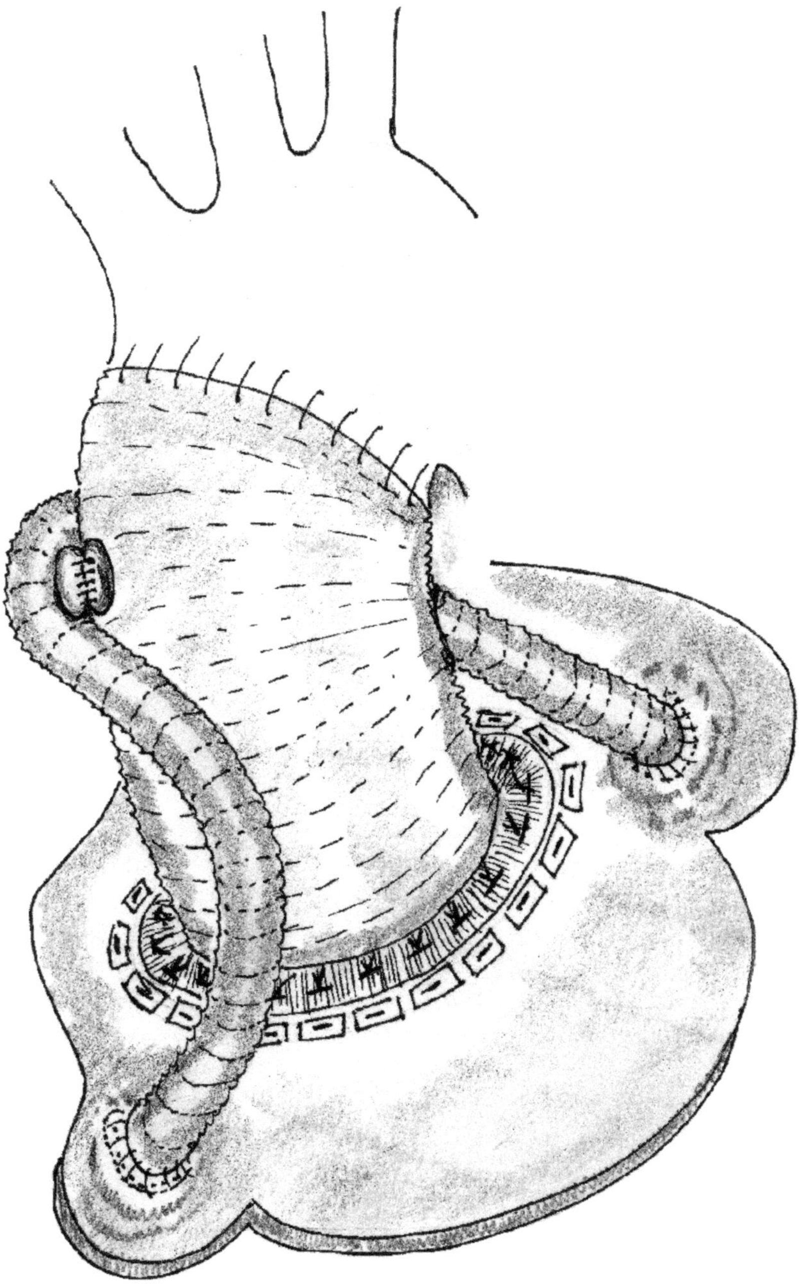

Figure 4. Cabrol procedure.

due to stenosis, thrombosis, and occlusion of the longer interposition graft, several modifications of this classic technique have been developed to mitigate these problems [37, 38]. There are three alternatives: an interposition graft can be anastomosed conjointly to coronary ostia; two small interposition grafts can be anastomosed between each coronary ostium and aortic graft separately; one coronary ostium can be anastomosed directly and the second ostium is anastomosed with a separate interposition graft to the aortic graft.

The Flanged technique prevents anastomotic difficulties of the proximal end of the composite graft, bleeding or dehiscence at the annular anastomosis (**Figure 5**). This technique provides the continuance of the flexibility and elasticity of the proximal end of the composite graft [39]. This method may be the best alternative for tailoring the aortic root in all aortic root pathologies, especially in patients with a small aortic root requiring posterior annular enlargement, calcified aortic annulus, aortic root abscess, or subannular defects. The length of the flange (1–3 cm long)

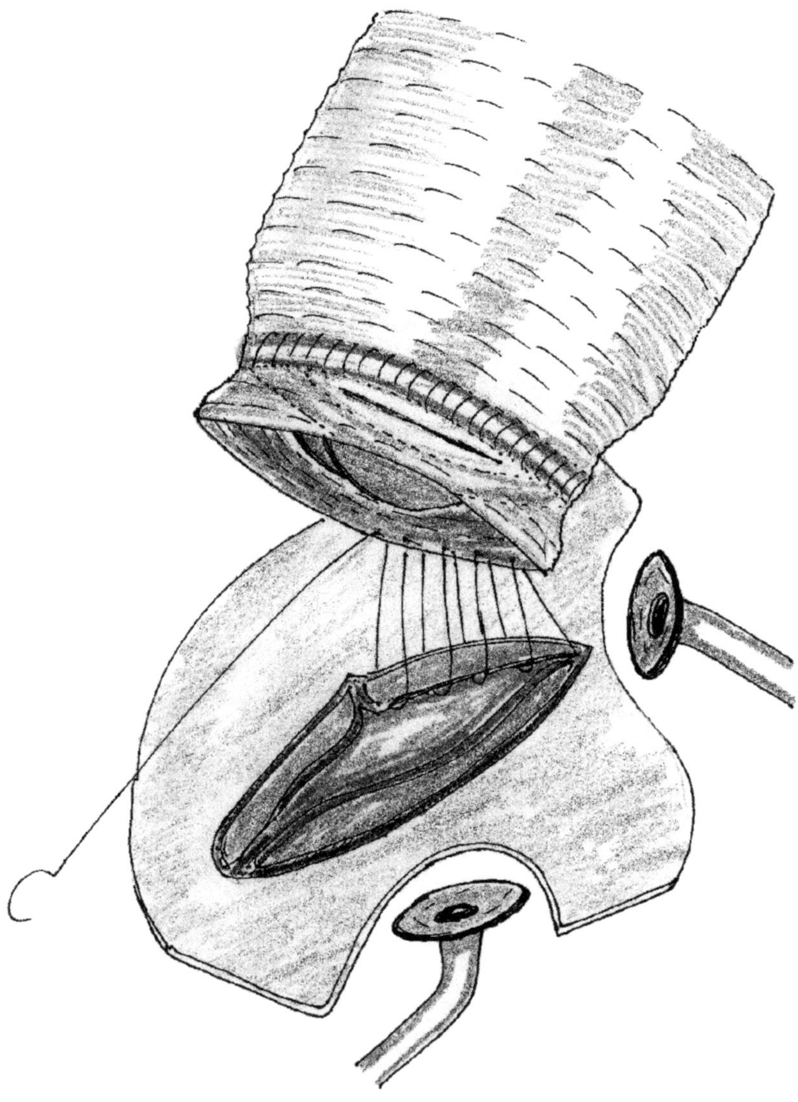

Figure 5. Flanged technique.

is adjusted depending on these procedures. The flange of the composite graft is implanted to the aortic annulus, where remained 3–5 mm aortic valve and the ascending aortic tissues are used as a double-sided strip (the free end of the tubular graft is interposed between these tissues) to prevent surgical bleeding and late pseudoaneurysm. In nondestroyed aortic annulus, sequential pledgeted mattress sutures can be incorporated to prevent postoperative bleeding through inter-sutures gaps. The newly created pseudosinusal tubular graft is the main preventive maneuver of this technique against stretching or kinking of the button anastomosis. The distal anastomosis of the composite tubular graft is performed in the same way as in the modified Bentall procedures.

The biologic Bentall technique with tissue composite graft provides an excellent hemodynamic profile similar to the native aortic root, very low transvalvular gradient, no anticoagulation, and very low risk of infection; however, the main disadvantage is structural degeneration. *Allograft* implantation is a reliable solution for the total ARR instead of prosthetic composite conduit options. The main indications are active destructive aortic valve endocarditis with root abscess, small aortic root in older patients, and contraindications against anticoagulation. But the use of allografts is infrequent because of limited availability of donors and the larger size roots. The root replacement technique has several advantages such as no distortion of the commissural positions, no asymmetry for the size mismatch, and the total exclusion of the native root pathology. In the case of a need of a patch or tissue below the aortic annulus, the mitral anterior leaflet of the allograft is also trimmed at this stage. Resection of the native aortic root with preparation of coronary buttons is similar in the Bentall procedure. *Xenograft* is a useful option for biologic Bentall because of the large availability of different sizes, improved durability, stentless structure, and reduced cost. Implantation of xenografts is very similar to aortic allograft [40].

The Ross technique is based on transferring the pulmonary root to the aortic position and the replacement of the pulmonary root with a pulmonary allograft or stentless porcine roots [41]. The pulmonary root can be an optimum substitute to the native aortic root, with a similar physiology and hemodynamic profile. The size difference between aortic and pulmonary annulus should not be more 2 mm, otherwise the diameter of the dilated aortic annulus should be reduced. The main advantages of the Ross technique are resistance to infection, no need for anticoagulation, and capability for somatic growth. However, the technical complexity of the operation and the risk of reintervention of the biologic grafts have limited widespread usage of the Ross procedure [42].

9.2. Total aortic root replacement with aortic valve sparing procedures

Aortic root pathologies with normal anatomic structure of the aortic leaflets causing significant aortic regurgitation are the primary indication for sparing aortic valve with/without aortic valve repair during the total ARR. Aortic valve sparing procedures allow avoidance of anticoagulation, prosthetic material, and postoperative transvalvular gradient. There are two major techniques with own advantages and disadvantages. The remodeling technique is preferred if any annular stabilization is not necessary, while the reimplantation technique is essential if annular stabilization is inevitable. The proximal anastomosis is completely different from valvular composite graft procedures, but coronary and distal anastomoses have similar surgical technical details to the modified Bentall procedure.

The remodeling technique (Yacoub procedure) does not touch the aortic annulus and/or subannular area (**Figure 6**). The ascending aorta is transected 2 cm above the sinotubular junction and then three sinuses of Valsalva are resected, leaving approximately 5 mm of aortic wall above the annulus for suturing of the tubular graft. The three commissures are hung up until the aortic

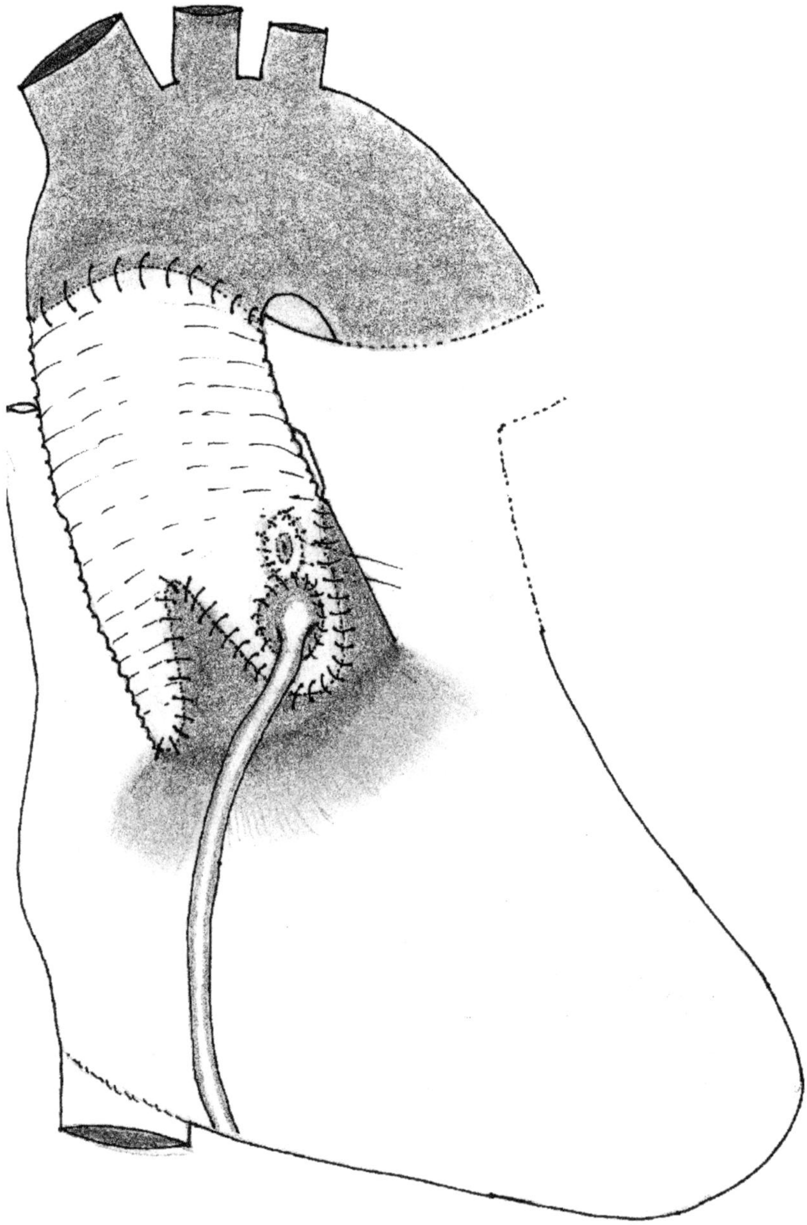

Figure 6. Remodeling technique (Yacoub).

http://dx.doi.org/10.5772/66963

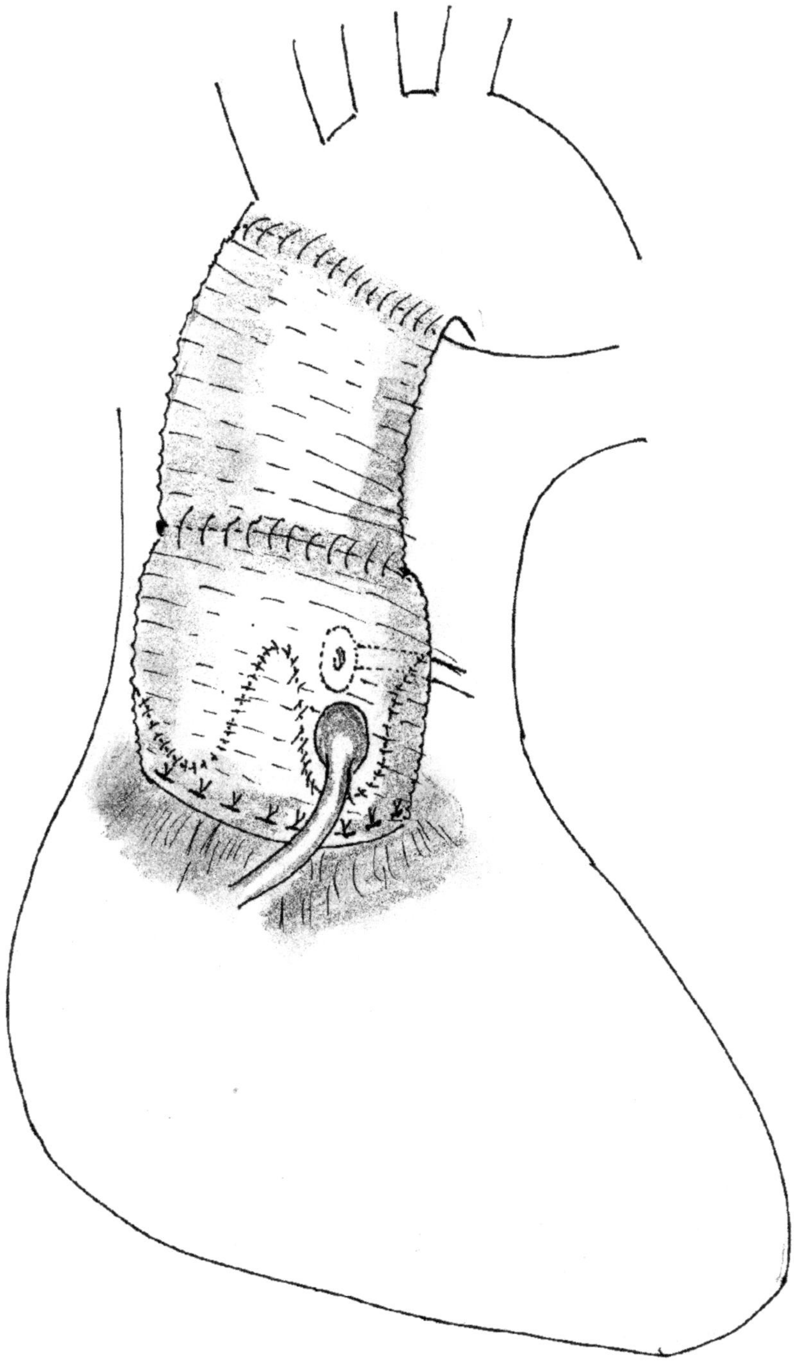

Figure 7. Reimplantation technique (David V).

leaflets coapt, and then appropriate sizing is performed to select the suitable graft. The stentless valve seizer is the easiest way to measure the annular diameter, and the number of seizer is the true graft size when it fills the aortic annulus. Three commissures are marked on the tubular graft and it is tailored to make three neo aortic sinuses, and their heights should be equal to the diameter of the graft. The graft with three tongues is sutured to the aortic wall at the annulus.

The reimplantation technique (David-V procedure) is useful for annular stabilization (**Figure 7**). The resection of the aortic root is similar to the remodeling technique, except graft preparing and suturing. If the ascending aorta dilatation causes aortic regurgitation with normal aortic annulus, the graft size must be equal to the annular diameter. In all other situations with aortic annular dilatation, the graft size should be decided very carefully. Because the straight graft causes native aortic valve deterioration, pseudosinuses are essential for avoidance of late valve degeneration. The larger graft is preferred for neo aortic root with neo pseudosinuses and the smaller graft is used for neo ascending aorta. To measure and decide the appropriate proximal tubular graft size, intra- or supra-annular seizers for stented bioprosthetic valves can be used [43]. If an *intra-annular seizer* is used, the appropriate graft size must be equal to the number of seizer (= inner diameter) + 5–6 mm. If a *supra-annular seizer* is used, the seizer is placed onto the aortic annulus and the base of three trigons should be visible through the supra-annular seizer. The appropriate graft size must be the number of seizer (= inner diameter) + 1–2 mm. When Valsalva graft is used for the reimplantation technique the graft size must be equal the height of the NCC-LCC commissure, which is equal to the external diameter of the sinotubular junction [44]. All mattress sutures with or without pledgets are passed from the inside of the left ventricle to the outside just below the aortic valve and then through the base of the graft and tied. That achieves annular reduction in patients with annular dilatation. The other important step is creating the correct position and height of commissures within the graft, which is the main mechanism to prevent leaflet prolapses and to secure competence of the aortic valve. After three placement sutures are tied, the aortic wall in each sinus is sutured continuously to the inside of the graft. The coronary artery reimplantations are performed by using the same procedure as described for the total ARR. The second smaller graft is anastomosed to the first graft, which helps to build a neo sinotubular junction and the crown-shaped aortic annulus. The key point during the anastomosis of both grafts together is to take the equal distance from both grafts for each bite at the commissural levels and longer from the proximal graft between commissures. This maneuver narrows intercommissural distance, which has been created by the larger proximal graft, to create an equal ring as a reduced annular ring [45].

9.3. Subtotal aortic root replacement procedures

These techniques are subtypes of the standard remodeling technique and popularized to avoid either a total composite or aortic valve sparing root replacement procedure. The aortic root seems more or less intact, and may distort aortic valve functions. Subtotal aortic root remodeling techniques can be preferred if all three sinuses are not involved without an aortic annular dilatation. Significant aortic annular dilatation requiring annular fixation is a contraindication for these approaches. Another indication is supravalvular stenosis, which can be congenital or acquired, and the repair option of this pathology depends on its involvement: single [46], double [47], or triple [48] sinus replacement. Isolated sinusal involvement usually affects NCS, especially in a bicuspid aortic valve. Aortic root enlargement is not diffuse and both coronary sinuses seem normal. The other rare pathology is restricted aortic dissection with/without involving the ascending aorta and chronic healing surrounds the dissection tear. The affected sinus can be replaced with a patch or with prosthetic tubular graft having a tongue-shape extension. If ascending aorta replacement is not necessary, a Dacron patch is tailored as a new sinus and sutured to the annulus of the resected sinus of Valsalva. The shape of the patch should be appropriate to the sinus, but the width should be <10 mm more than the diameter between two commissures and the height <10 mm more than the diameter from the annulus to the sinotubular junction. Subtotal root remodeling on the two sinuses can be chosen for acute aortic dissection without left coronary ostial involvement if aortic root dilatation is not greater than 35 mm, which can prevent the reimplantation of the left coronary ostium. On the contrary, if both coronary sinuses are involved or the presence of aortic annular dilatation requires aortic annular stabilization, any total ARR is more meaningful.

9.4. Sinus of Valsalva aneurysm repair techniques

Repair is recommended for ruptured aneurysms, significant aortic valve regurgitation, associated intracardiac abnormalities, or symptomatic unruptured or enlarging aneurysm. Rupture of sinus of Valsalva aneurysm is a life-threatening complication and requires immediate surgical or interventional closure. Surgical closure is the gold standard treatment, but percutaneous closure can be chosen in very sick patients [49]. Different surgical approaches can be used: transaortic, double-chamber, or involved chamber. The transaortic approach is used for isolated sinus of Valsalva aneurysm with/without aortic regurgitation, especially in unruptured cases. The double-chamber approach is chosen mostly in ruptured aneurysms because of closing defect from both sides or the presence of any intracardiac pathology [50]. The last approach is used very seldom because of possible bacterial colonization or thrombus formation inside the aneurysm, or recurrent fistula formation or rupture of aneurysmal sac. The goals of repair are removing the aneurysmal sac, closing the defect primary or with a patch or with valve replacement, and repairing any associated defects. Patch closure at the aortic end is the most preferred technique, which minimizes aortic leaflet distortion, with/without a concomitant surgery for aortic valve repair.

9.5. The extensive aortic root replacement technique

Aortic root abscess continues to challenge cardiovascular surgeons, because uncontrolled aortic root abscess can manifest itself as a burrowing pathology destroying the whole aortic annulus and extending proximally into the left ventricular outflow tract, a cardiac fistula or a rupture into a cardiac chamber, a pseudoaneurysm, or an arrhythmia leading to hemodynamic instability. Early and extensive surgical intervention of aortic root abscesses is essential, and the complexity of the surgical treatment ranges from partial resection of the aortic annulus and surrounding tissues to radical removal of the base of the heart—including the entire aortic root, the intervalvular fibrous body, and part of the interventricular septum.

The extensive ARR technique is the only option to rebuild the left ventricular outflow tract due to the reconstruction of the neo aortoventricular continuity in the isolated aortic root abscess. The flanged technique with the elongated tubular graft below the prosthetic valve is the best option for solving this life-threatening sequel and reconstructing the aortic root [51]. A larger (3 cm) segment of the proximal end of the tubular graft is implanted in a circular manner with 2–0 interrupted sutures supported by large Teflon pledgets placed subannularly on healthy tissue at the native left ventricular outflow tract. Both ends of the sutures are passed through the proximal free end of the flanged portion of the conduit in order to use that part as a strip between knots and the myocardial aortic wall.

Author details

Kaan Kırali[1,2]* and Deniz Günay[1]

*Address all correspondence to: imkbkirali@yahoo.com

1 Deptatrment of Cardiovascular Surgery, Kartal Kosuyolu YI Education and Research Hospital, Istanbul, Turkey

2 Deptartment of Cardiovascular Surgery, Faculty of Medicine, University of Sakarya, Sakarya, Turkey

References

[1] Lang RM, Badano LP, Mor-Avi V, Afilalo J, Armstrong A, Ernande L, Flachskampf FA, Foster E, Goldstein SA, Kuznetsova T, Lancellotti P, Muraru D, Picard MH, Rietzschel ER, Rudski L, Spencer KT, Tsang W, Voigt JU. Recommendations for cardiac chamber quantification by echocardiography in adults: An update from the American Society of Echocardiography and the European Association of Cardiovascular Imaging. J Am Soc Echocardiogr 2015;28(1):1–39.

[2] Evangelista A, Flachskampf FA, Erbel R, Antonini-Canterin F, Vlachopoulos C, Rocchi G, Sicari R, Nihoyannopoulos P, Zamorano J. Echocardiography in aortic diseases: EAE recommendations for clinical practice. Eur J Echocardiogr 2010;11(8):645–658.

[3] Hal-Ali R, Marom G, Zekry SB, Rosenfeld M, Raanani E. A general three-dimensional parametric geometry of the native aortic valve and root for biomechanical modeling. J Biomech 2012;45(14):2392–2397.

[4] Khelil N, Sleilaty G, Palladino M, Fouda M, Escande R, Debauchez M, Di Centa I, Lansac E. Surgical anatomy of the aortic annulus: Landmarks for external annuloplasty in aortic valve repair. Ann Thorac Surg 2015;99(4):1220–1227.

[5] Choo SJ, McRae G, Olomon JP, St George G, Davis W, Burleson-Bowles CL, Pang D, Luo HH, Vavra D, Cheung DT, Oury JH, Duran CM. Aortic root geometry: Pattern of differences between leaflets and sinuses of Valsalva. J Heart Valve Dis 1999;8(4):407–415.

[6] Contino M, Mangini A, Lemma MG, Romagnoni C, Zerbi P, Gelpi G, Antona C. A geometric approach to aortic root surgical anatomy. Eur J Cardiothorac Surg 2016;49(1):93–100.

[7] Martin M, Sievers HH. Heart valve macro-and microstructure. Philos Trans R Soc Lond B Biol Sci (2007); 362(1484):1421–1436.

[8] Rabkin SW. Accentuating and opposing factors leading to development of thoracic aortic aneurysms not due to genetic or inherited conditions. Front Cardiovasc Med 2015;2:21.

[9] Toumpoulis IK, Oxford JT, Cowan DB, Anagnostopoulus CE, Rokkas CK, Chamogeorgakis TP, Angouras DC, Shemin RJ, Navab M, Ericsson M, Federman M, Levitsky S, McCully JD. Differential expression of collagen type V and XI α-1 in human ascending thoracic aortic aneurysms. Ann Thorac Surg 2009;88(2):506–513.

[10] Huusko T, Salonurmi T, Taskinen P, Liinamaa J, Juvonen T, Pääkkö P, Savolainen M, Kakko S. Elevated messenger RNA expression and plasma protein levels of osteopontin and matrix metalloproteinase types 2 and 9 in patients with ascending aortic aneurysms. J Thorac Cardiovasc Surg 2013;145(4):1117–1123.

[11] Jackson V, Olsson T, Kurtovic S, Folkersen L, Paloschi V, Wågsäter D, Franco-Cereceda A, Ericsson M. Matrix metalloproteinase 14 and 19 expression is associated with thoracic aortic aneurysms. J Thorac Cardiovasc Surg 2012;144(2):459–466.

[12] Zhang L, Liao MF, Tian L, Zou SL, Lu QS, Bao JM. Overexpression of interleukin-1β and interferon-γ in type I thoracic aortic dissections and ascending thoracic aortic aneurysms: Possible correlation with matrix metalloproteinase-9 expression and apoptosis of aortic media cells. Eur J Cardiothorac Surg 2011;40(1):17–22.

[13] Gillis E, Van Laer L, Loeys BL. Genetics of thoracic aortic aneurysm: at the crossroad of transforming growth factor-β signaling and vascular smooth muscle cell contractility. Circ Res 2013;113(3):327–340.

[14] Verma S, Siu SC. Aortic dilatation in patients with bicuspid aortic valve. N Engl J Med 2014;370(20):1920–1929.

[15] Fazel SS, Mallidi HR, Lee RS,. The aortopathy of bicuspid aortic valve disease has distinctive patterns and usually involves the transverse aortic arch. J Thorac Cardiovasc Surg 2008;135(4):901–907.

[16] Kirali K, Guler M, Daglar B, Yakut N, Mansuroglu D, Balkanay M, Berki T, Gürbüz A, Isık O, Yakut C. Surgical repair in ruptured congenital sinus of Valsalva aneurysms: A 13-year experience. J Heart Valve Dis 1999;8(4):424–429.

[17] Kırali K, Yakut N, Güler M, Mansuroğlu D, Ömeroğlu S, Akıncı E, Gürbüz A, Yakut C. Surgical treatment of siblings with Marfan syndrome. Asian Cardiovasc Thorac Ann 1999;7(2):138–141.

[18] Erbel R, Aboyans V, Boileau C, Bossone E, Bartolomes RD, Eggebrecht H, Evangelista A, Falk V, Frank H, Gaemperli O, Grabenwöger M, Haverich A, ıung B, Manolis AJ, Meijboom F, Nienaber CA, Roffi M, Rousseau H, Sechtem U, Sirnes PA, von Allmen RS, Vrints CJM. 2014 ESC Guidelines on the diagnosis and treatment of aortic diseases. The

task force for the diagnosis and treatment of aortic diseases of the European Society of Cardiology (ESC). Eur Heart J 2014;35,:2873–2926.

[19] Garg V, Ouzounian M, Peterson MD. Advances in aortic disease management: A year in review. Curr Opin cardiol 2016;31(2):127–131.

[20] Michielon G, Salvador L, Da Col U, Valfrè C. Modified button-Bentall operation for aortic root replacement: The miniskirt technique. Ann Thorac Surg 2001;72:S1059–1064.

[21] Suzuki A, Amano J, Tanaka H, Sakamoto T, Sunamori M. Surgical consideration of aortitis involving the aortic root. Circulation 1989;80(3):I222–232.

[22] Yakut C. A new modified Bentall procedure: The flanged technique. Ann Thorac Surg 2001;71(6):2050–2052.

[23] De Paulis R, De Matteis GM, Nardi P, Scaffa R, Colella DF, Chiarello L. A new aortic Dacron conduit for surgical treatment of aortic root pathology. Ital Heart J 2000;1(7):457–463.

[24] Kırali K. Technique of awake off-pump coronary artery bypass grafting. In: Raja SG, Amrani M, editors. Off-pump Coronary Artery Bypass Grafting. New York: Nova Science Publishers Inc; 2012, pp. 175–211.

[25] Chakravarthy M, Jawali V, Patil TA, Jayaprakash K, Kolar S, Joseph G, Das JK, Maheswari U, Sudhakar N. Conscious cardiac surgery with cardiopulmonary bypass using thoracic epidural anesthesia without endotracheal general anesthesia. J Cardiothorac Vasc Anesth 2005;19(3):300–305.

[26] Bottio T, Bisleri G, Piccoli P, Negri A, Manzato A, Muneretto C. Heart valve surgery in a very high-risk population: A preliminary experience in awake patients. J Heart Valve Dis 2007;16(2):187–194.

[27] Porizka M, Stritesky M, Semrad M, Dobias M, Dohnalova A, Korinek J. Standard blood flow rates of cardiopulmonary bypass are adequate in awake on-pump cardiac surgery. Eur J Cardiothorac Surg 2011;39(4):442–450.

[28] Kırali K, Kayalar N, Özen Y, Sareyyüpoğlu B, Güzelmeriç F, Koçak T, Yakut C. Reversed-J inferior versus full median sternotomy: Which is better for awake coronary bypass surgery. J Card Surg 2005;20(5):463–468.

[29] Lentini S, Specchia L, Nicolardi S, Mangia F, Rasovic O, Di Eusanio G, Gregorini R. Surgery of the ascending aorta with or without combined procedures through an upper ministernotomy: Outcomes of a series of more than 100 patients. Ann Thorac Cardiovasc Surg 2006;22(1):44–48.

[30] Ozer T, Akbulut M, Altas O, Mataraci I, Tuncer MA, Kirali MK. Partial upper sternotomy for concomitant with ascendant aorta replacement or isolated aortic valve implantation (abstract). Aortic Symposium, 2016, May 12–13. New York, NY, USA.

[31] Russo MJ, Gnezda J, Merlo A, Johnson EM, Hashmi M, Raman J. The arrowhead ministernotomy with rigid sternal plate fixation: A minimally invasive approach for surgery of the ascending aorta and aortic root. Minim Invasive Surg 2014, 681371.

[32] Özer T, Altaş Ö, Sarıkaya S, Özen Y, Yerlikhan EO, Günay D, Hançer H, Kırali K. Double reverse incisions make aortic valve surgery lesser invasive (abstract). 12th International Congress of Update in Cardiology and Cardiovascular Surgery, 2016, March 10–13. Belek, Antalya, Turkey.

[33] Tuncer A, Tuncer EY, Polat A, Mataracı İ, Keleş C, Alsalehi S, Boyacıoğlu K, Kara İ, Kırali K. Axillary artery cannulation in ascending aortic pathologies. Turkish J Thorac Cardiovasc Surg 2011;19(4):539–544.

[34] Kırali K. Surgical strategy in aortic root aneurysms: Modified Bentall-aortic valve sparing surgery. Turkiye Klinikleri J Cardiovasc Surg-Special Topics 2012;4(1):7–17.

[35] Copeland JG 3d, Rosado LJ, Snyder SL. New technique for improving hemostasis in aortic root replacement with composite graft. Ann Thorac Surg 1993;55(4):1027–1029.

[36] Chen LW, Dai XF, Wu XJ. A modified composite valve Dacron graft for prevention of postoperative bleeding from the proximal anastomosis after Bentall procedure. Ann Thorac Surg 2009;88(5):1705–1707.

[37] Kourliouros A, Soni M, Rasoli S, Grapsa J, Nihoyannopoulos P, O'Regan D, Athanasiou T. Evolution and current applications of the Cabrol procedure and its modifications. Ann Thorac Surg 2011;91(5):1636–1641.

[38] Ziganshin BA, Williams FE, Tranquilli M, Elefteriades JA. Midterm experience with modified Cabrol procedure: Safe and durable for complex aortic root replacement. J Thorac Cardiovasc Surg 2014;147(4):1233–1239.

[39] Kırali K, Mansuroğlu D, Ömeroğlu SN, Erentuğ V, Mataracı I, Ipek G, Akıncı E, Işık Ö, Yakut C. Five-year experience in aortic root replacement with the flanged composite graft. Ann Thorac Surg 2002;73(4):1130–1137.

[40] Yıldırım T, Güler M, Kırali K, Ömeroğlu SN, Eren E, Toker ME, Balkanay M, Dağlar B, Akıncı E, İpek G, Yakut C. Stentless bioprostheses in aortic root surgery: Mid-term results. Turk Kardiyol Dern Ars 2000;28(10):630–634.

[41] Juthier F, Vincentelli A, Hysi I, Pinçon C, Rousse N, Banfi C, Prat A. Stentless porcine bioprosthesis in pulmonary position after Ross procedure: Midterm results. Ann Thorac Surg 2015;99(4):1255–1259.

[42] Reece TB, Welke KF, O'Brien S, Grau-Sepulveda MV, Grover FL, Gammie JS. Rethinking the Ross procedure in adults. Ann Thorac Surg 2014;97(1):175–181.

[43] Kırali K, Sarıkaya S, Elibol A, Göçer S, Özer T, Altaş Ö, Ünal ÜS, Şişmanoğlu M. Aortic root replacement with the reimplantation procedure: Simplifying the sizing of tubular graft (abstract). 20th Annual Meeting for Asian Society for Cardiovascular and Thoracic Surgery, 2012, March 7-12. Bali, Indonesia.

[44] de Kerchove L, Boodhwani M, Glineur D, Noirhomme P, El Khoury G. A new simple and objective method for graft sizing in valve-sparing root replacement using the reimplantation technique. Ann Thorac Surg 2011;92(2):749–751.

[45] Kırali K, Altas O, Ozer T, Gunay D, Hancer H, Sarikaya S, Ozen Y. David-V aortic valve sparing procedure: Mid-ter results (abstract). Aortic Symposium 2016. 2016, May 12–13. New York, NY, USA.

[46] Dağlar B, Kırali K, Yakut N, Tuncer A, Balkanay M, İpek G, Akıncı E, Yakut C. The surgical repair of congenital supravalvular aortic stenosis by single sinus aortoplasty technique: Mid-long term results. Turkish J Thorac Cardiovasc Surg 1999;7(3):223–228.

[47] Katayama A, Uchida N, Sutoh M, Sueda T. Partial root remodeling on the two sinuses for acute type a aortic dissection with right coronary arterial dissection. Ann Vasc Dis 2013;6(3):666–669.

[48] Yokoyama S, Nagato H, Yoshida Y, Nagasaka S, Kaneda K, Nishiwaki N. Novel three-sinus enlargement technique for supravalvular aortic stenosis without aortic transection. J Cardiothorac Surg 2016;11(4), doi: 10.1186/s13019-016-0403-5.

[49] Kuriakose EM, Bhatla P, McElhinney DB. Comparison of reported outcomes with percutaneous versus surgical closure of ruptured sinus of Valsalva aneurysm. Am J Cardiol 2015;115(3):39392–39398.

[50] Sarıkaya S, Adademir T, Elibol A, Büyükbayrak F, Onk A, Kırali K. Surgery for ruptured sinus of Valsalva aneurysm: 25-year experience with 55 patients. Eur J Cardio-Thorac Surg 2013;43(3):591–596.

[51] Kırali K, Sarikaya S, Ozen Y, Sacli H, Basaran E, Yerlikhan OA, Aydın E, Rabus MB. Surgery for aortic root abscess: 15-year experience. Tex Heart Inst J 2016;43(1):20–28.

Section 3

Aortic Arch Aneuryms

Chapter 3

Experimental and Numerical Study of the Flow Dynamics in Treatment Approaches for Aortic Arch Aneurysms

Asaph Nardi, Barak Even-Chen and Idit Avrahami

Additional information is available at the end of the chapter

http://dx.doi.org/10.5772/66976

Abstract

Aortic arch aneurysm is a complex aortic pathology which affects one or more aortic arch vessels. In this chapter, we explore the hemodynamic behavior of the aortic arch in aneurysmatic and treated cases with three currently available treatment approaches: surgery graft, hybrid stent-graft and chimney stent-graft. The analysis included time-dependent experimental and numerical models of aneurysmatic arch and of the surgery, hybrid and chimney endovascular techniques. Dimensions of the models are based on typical anatomy, and boundary conditions are based on typical physiological flow. Flexible and transparent experimental models were used on a mock circulation in vitro experimental system to allow both visualization and time-dependent flow and pressure measurements. The simulations used computational fluid dynamics (CFD) methods to delineate the time-dependent flow dynamics in the four geometric models. Results of velocity vectors, flow patterns, pressure and wall shear stress distributions are presented. Both the numerical and experimental results agree on the poor hemodynamics of the aortic arch aneurysm and present the hemodynamic advantages of the surgery technique, implying the possible advantage of fenestrated stent-graft for the aortic arch. Out of the two minimally invasive procedures, the hybrid procedure clearly exhibits better hemodynamic performances. The chimney graft technique is based on off-the-shelf devices; thus, it is low in cost and requires less pre-operation preparations. However, it is associated with higher risks for complications, such as endoleaks and stroke. This chapter may give some insight into the hemodynamic characteristics of the different procedures.

Keywords: thoraces aortic aneurysm, endovascular repair, stent-graft, CFD, in vitro visualization

1. Introduction

Aortic arch aneurysm is a rare condition of aortic aneurysm with relatively high fatal risk for fast enlargement and rapture [1–3]. Aortic arch aneurysms or thoracoabdominal aneurysm (that involves large portions of the aorta) are considered complex aortic pathologies require coverage of one or more aortic arch vessels (as sketched, for example, in **Figure 1a**) and are usually repaired using total vessel replacement via open surgery (as sketched in **Figure 1b**).

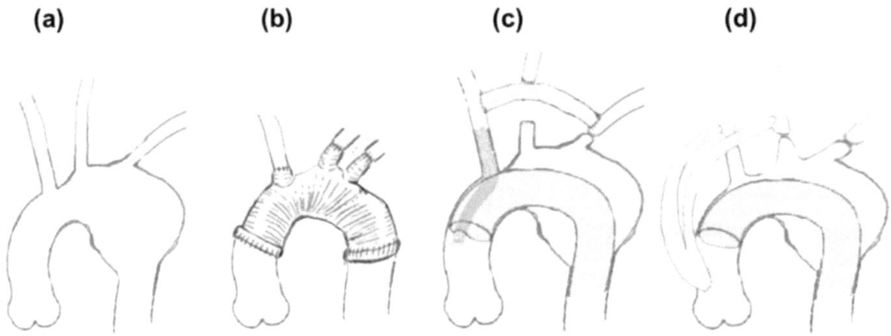

Figure 1. Schematic illustrations of aortic arch with: (a) aneurysm; (b) surgery graft; (c) chimney SG and (d) hybrid graft.

The introduction of endovascular aneurysm repair (EVAR) offers an attractive minimally invasive alternative for diseases of the aortic aorta. This technology has advanced to treat more complicated cases of aneurysm thanks to advances in imaging and materials technology. The surgical procedure for aortic arch replacement is considered one of the most challenging cardiac surgeries, which often requires a combination of median sternotomy and lateral thoracotomy and usually requires aortic cross-clamping and hypothermic circulatory arrest. It is a highly complex operation which carries a substantial risk of morbidity and mortality [4, 5]. The EVAR alternative, on the other hand, is a procedure that requires only small incisions in the groin, local anesthesia and without interrupting blood flow. EVAR procedures are associated with a lower morbidity and mortality compared to open repair technique [6–8].

However, EVAR techniques face a major challenge in the repair of the aortic arch, which is to maintain blood flow to the side branches in the sealing zone of the graft [9]. Since this condition is relatively rare and complicated, no standard clinically approved device was introduced yet and most of the reported clinical solutions to overcome this challenge are patient specific in house combination that can fall into one of the two major approach classifications: (i) the graft procedures using fenestrations or chimney technique (e.g., chimney of innominate artery, as sketched in **Figure 1c**), or (ii) the total hybrid debranching procedures (**Figure 1d**) [10].

In the chimney graft technique [7, 11, 12], a covered stent is placed parallel to the main aortic stent-graft, similar to a chimney, providing the necessary blood perfusion to the vital upper branches. In order to distribute the blood flow among the other upper branches, bypasses are also required between the side branches. For example, a bypass between the innominate artery (IA) and the left subclavian artery (LSA) and between the LSA and the left common carotid artery (LCCA), as shown in **Figure 1c**. The chimney graft technique allows the use of standard off-the-shelf covered stents for an emergency or immediate treatments of challenging aneurysms without sufficient neck, allowing an alternative to fenestrated stent-grafts in urgent cases [13].

In the hybrid total aortic arch debranching, a bifurcated Dacron graft is connected to the ascending aorta using a proximal end-to-side anastomosis [14–17]. The deployment of the endograft is done after bypassing the LSA as shown in **Figure 1d**.

Both approaches were proven to be technically feasible with high short-term technical success rate and relatively favorable rates of perioperative outcomes. Long-term outcomes remain undefined [12, 18–20]. The hybrid technique is considered to have better performance [21]; however, it uses custom-made devices associated with long manufacturing times and increased costs [22]. The chimney technique has the advantage of applying available off-the-shelf devices, being technically less complicated. However, in high-risk patients, it is associated with a relevant morbidity, mortality and reintervention rate. Therefore, it is often recommended only for patients not suitable for conventional aortic arch repair or emergency cases at present [23, 24].

In this study, we show the similarities between the numerical mesh and the visualization models, thus properly representing the case, while obtaining similar flow patterns and regimes.

2. Methods

2.1. Experimental models

Four silicone prototype models were procured by dipping, representing typical anatomical geometries of the four cases. A hybrid graft was manually fitted using Propoxy 20 as seen in **Figure 2a**, to modify the healthy case. **Figure 2b** displays the resulted hybrid model after being fitted with the hybrid graft and a placement of a bypass between the LCCA and LSA. Note the clipping of the LCCA and IA arteries at their connection point to the aortic arch according to surgery specs using silicone glue.

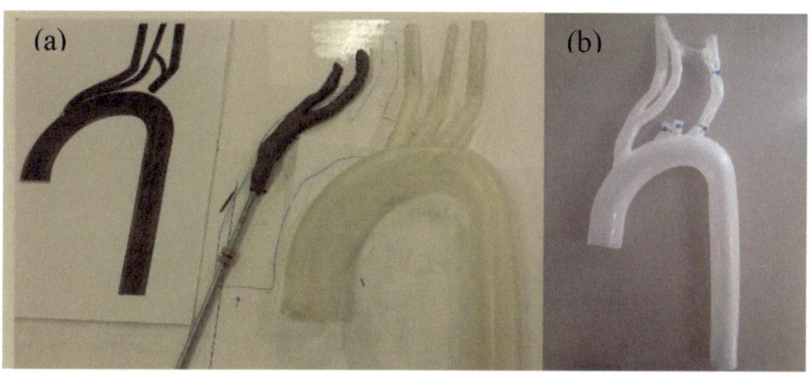

Figure 2. (a) Fitting the hybrid bypass mold to the real size model according to surgery specifications and (b) the resulted model.

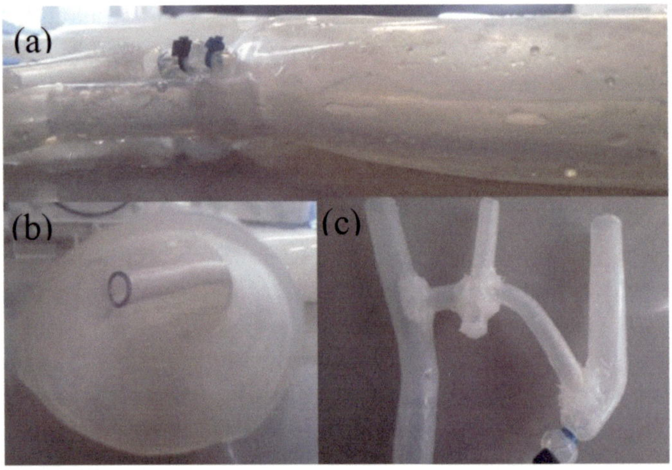

Figure 3. Remodeling the original model to match the chimney technique. Note the: (a) insertion of the stent graft into the Aortic arch and IA, (b) the permanent placement of the inner tube modeling the SG and (c) the connection of the LSA and LCCA arteries to the IA via a bypass.

Modifying a healthy case model to a chimney graft model was done, by inserting a 10-mm diameter tube—representing a stent-graft (SG) from the IA down to the aortic arch as seen in **Figure 3a**. In order to enable the insertion, the IA was cut and reconnected to the aortic arch. **Figure 3b** shows the permanent placement of the inner tube representing a SG. Note the bypass connection to the various arteries using an adhesive.

After gluing all of the models and bypasses, every model underwent a pressure test to insure no endoleaks. The hybrid model during visual sealing verification prior to a pressure test is seen in **Figure 4a** and during a pressure test in **Figure 4b**. Note the stream of water leaking from the bypasses connection to the LSA.

The four finalized models are seen in **Figure 5**.

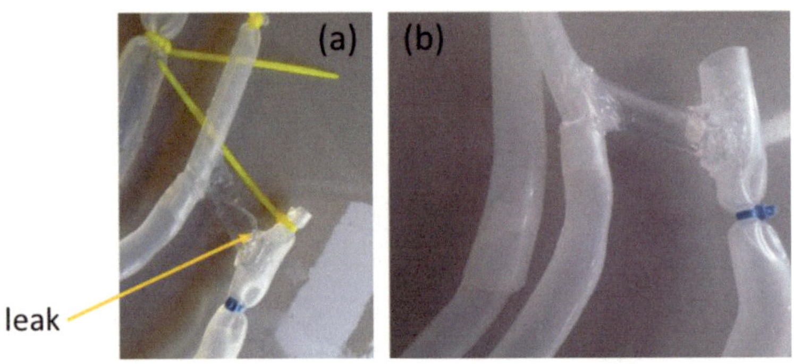

Figure 4. The hybrid model (a) during a pressure test. Note the leaking water stream at the bypasses connection point and (b) after fixing the leak.

http://dx.doi.org/10.5772/66976

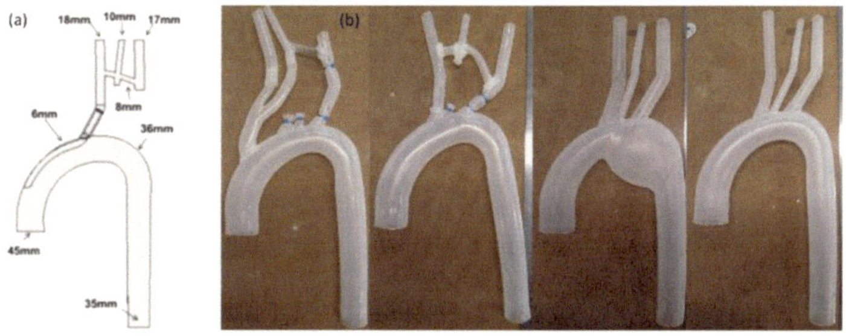

Figure 5. (a) Typical model dimensions and (b) the four silicone models.

2.2. Pulse duplicator flow loop and particle image set-up

An in vitro experimental set-up was utilized to create image aortic, graft and bypass flow. A pulse duplicator flow loop was constructed to generate pulsatile flow to mimic the physiological conditions of the arterial system using a positive displacement pump (enabler by hemo dynamics) as seen in **Figure 6a**. Each model was placed in turn into the system, where the aortic root was connected to a model of a three-leaflet aortic valve which was connected to a bubble trap and a pulse duplicator. A series of valves were placed at the IA, LSA, LCCA and descending aorta, respectively, to control pressure and flow rates as seen in **Figure 6b**. The mean inlet flow rate was set at 4 L/min at 60 beats per minute. Flow volume in the IA, LCCA and LSA was set to 0.4, 0.32 and 0.28 L/min, respectively, according to common physiological distribution rates. The IA, LCCA and LSA arteries were then reconnected to a reservoir.

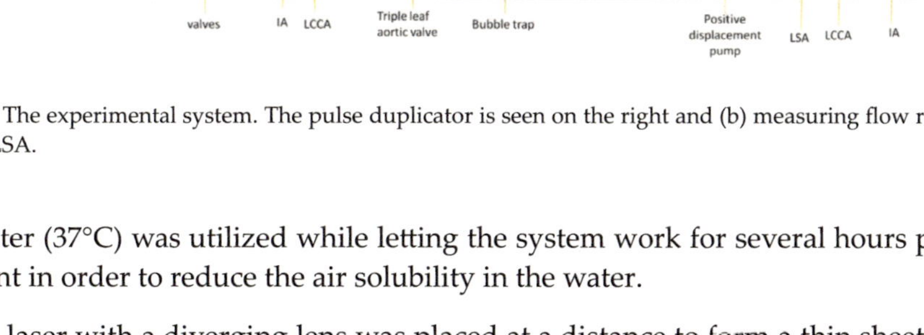

Figure 6. (a) The experimental system. The pulse duplicator is seen on the right and (b) measuring flow rates at the IA, LCCA and LSA.

Warm water (37°C) was utilized while letting the system work for several hours prior to the experiment in order to reduce the air solubility in the water.

A 532 nm laser with a diverging lens was placed at a distance to form a thin sheet of light. A high speed camera (Bonito, Allied vision technologies, Germany) was placed at a 90° angle beneath the model. Fluoresentric particles were then injected into the system, and videos and still shots were taken and analyzed.

2.3. Numerical analysis

The numerical model is fully described in previous publications [19] and is briefly described below. The numerical analysis included computational fluid dynamics (CFD) simulations of the time-dependent flow in models of the aneurysmatic arch and of the surgery, hybrid and chimney endovascular techniques (**Figure 7**), identical to the experimental models.

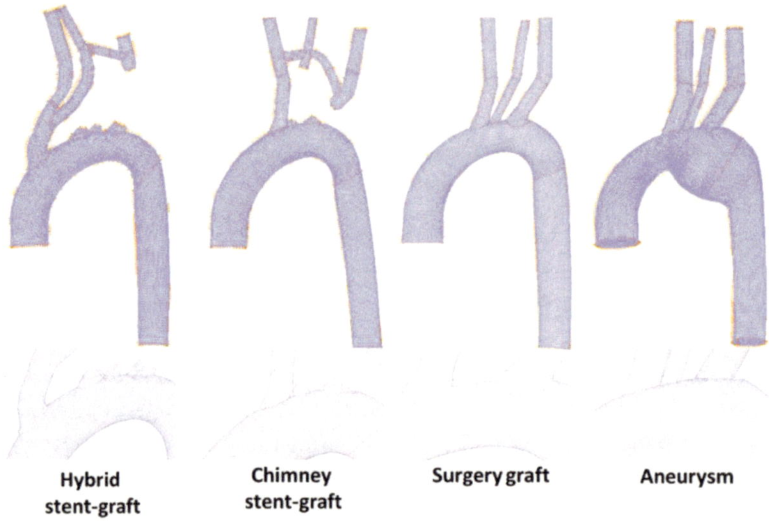

Figure 7. The four numerically meshed models (top—full models and bottom—magnified view).

The numerical model is fully detailed elsewhere [19] and will be presented here briefly. The model solves numerically the equations governing momentum and continuity in the fluid domain:

$$\begin{gathered} \nabla \cdot V = 0 \\ \rho \frac{DV}{Dt} = -\nabla p + \mu \nabla^2 V + \rho g \end{gathered} \tag{1}$$

where p is static pressure, t is time, **V** is the velocity vector, ρ and μ are density and dynamic viscosity of the fluid, respectively, and **g** is the vector of gravity. The flow was assumed laminar and the fluid was assumed homogenous, incompressible (with density $\rho = 1$ g/mL) and Newtonian.

In order to compare the numerical models with the experiments, the simulations used water (with viscosity $\mu = 1$ cP). In addition, simulations with blood ($\mu = 3.5$ cP) were also performed.

The boundary conditions were similar to those specified for the experimental apparatus. The time-dependent inlet aortic flow and outlet pressure are shown in **Figure 8a**. Flow distribution between branches outlets was imposed as described in **Figure 8b**.

The commercial software ADINA (ADINA R&D Inc., MA) was used to solve the set of fluid equations using the finite-element scheme. The numerical meshes consisted of 0.5–1 M tetrahedral elements each. For each case, a single cardiac cycle was analyzed with 10 time steps per cycle. Mesh and time-step validation test were performed as detailed in previous reports [19].

http://dx.doi.org/10.5772/66976

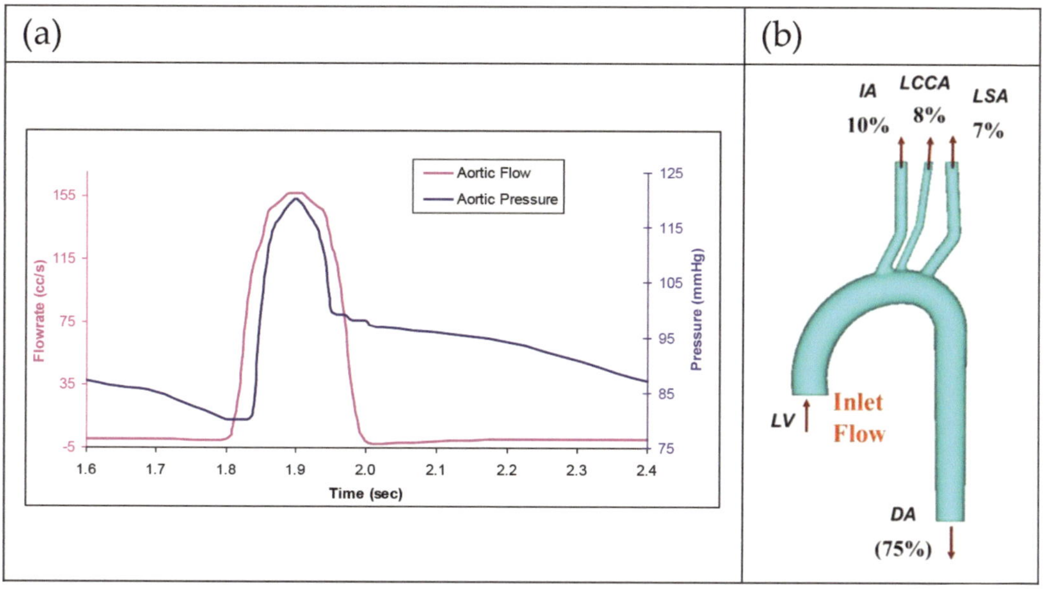

Figure 8. Boundary conditions of the numerical models: (a) inlet aortic flow and outlet pressure, as a function of time and (b) flow distribution between side branches (IA, innominate artery; LSA, left Subclavian artery; LCCA, left common carotid artery; DA, descending aorta).

3. Results

The resulted flow fields as calculated and visualized in the four cases are presented in **Figures 9–14**.

In the aneurysmatic case, three noticeable vortices are calculated (as seen in **Figure 9a**) and visualized (**Figure 9b**). In both methods, similar flow patterns dominant the flow field, including a

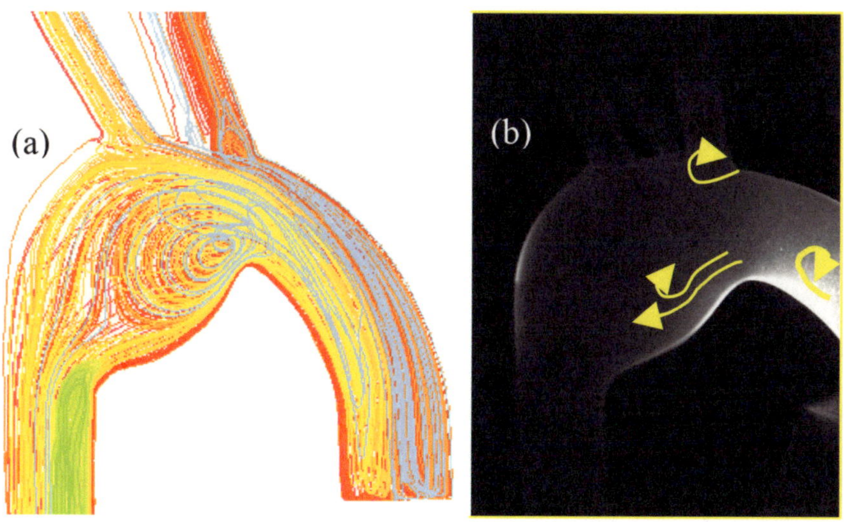

Figure 9. Flow patterns in the aneurysm case—(a) CFD particle trace and (b) visualization.

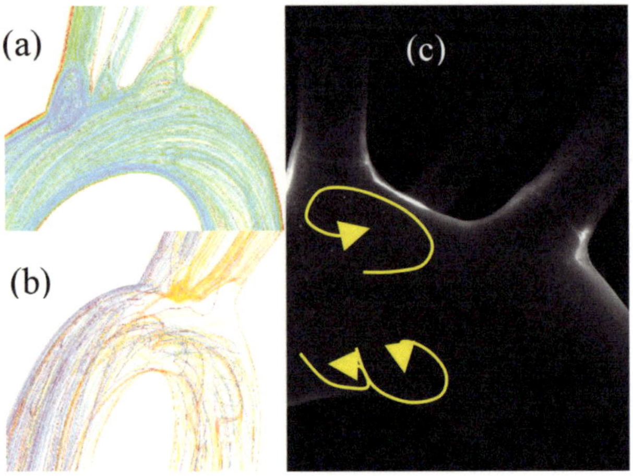

Figure 10. Flow patterns in the surgery graft. (a and b) CFD particle trace (c) visualization.

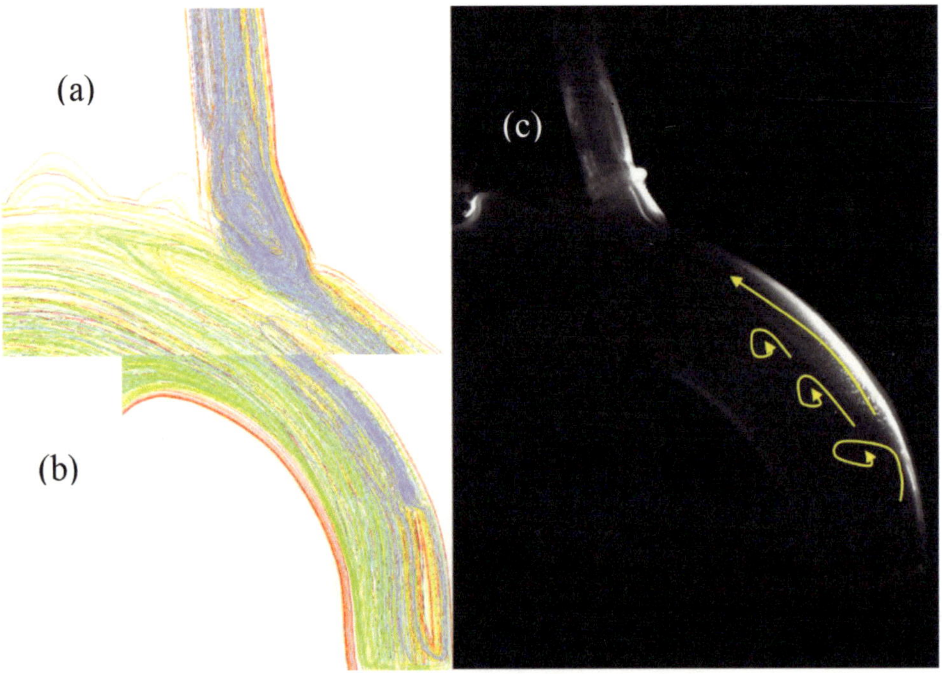

Figure 11. Flow patterns in the chimney graft (a) CFD particle trace at the IA branching (b) CFD particle trace in the aorta adjacent to the chimney graft (c) visualization.

single major vortex toward the center of the aneurysm accompanied by a shear layer between the vortex and the aneurysm wall. During diastole, a single vortex appears at the branching point of the IA with the aortic arch and a smaller vortex preceding the aneurysm.

Figure 10 shows flow patterns in the surgery graft case as calculated (a and b) and visualized (c). The branching arteries provoke vortices that form during the diastole. Helical flow starts near

http://dx.doi.org/10.5772/66976

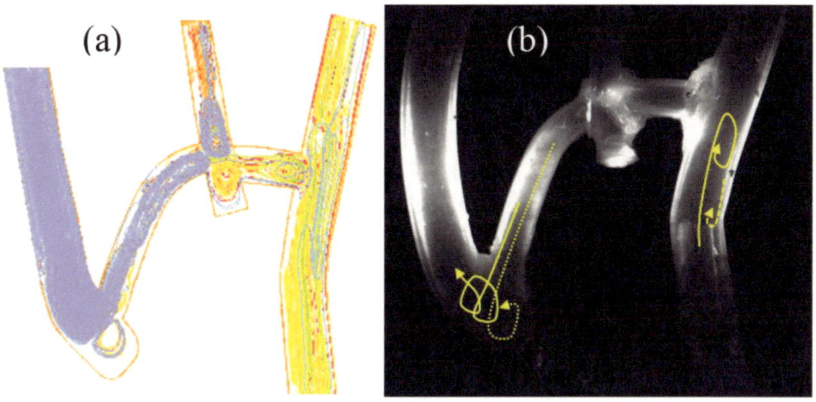

Figure 12. Flow patterns in the chimney bypass (a) CFD particle trace (b) visualization.

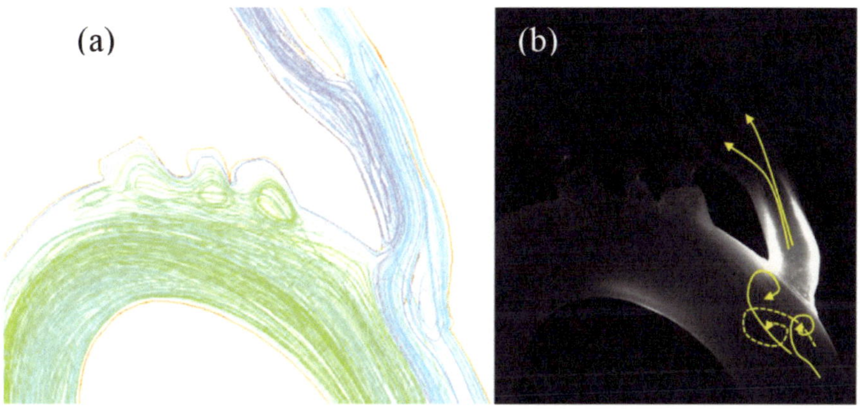

Figure 13. Hybrid graft (a) particle trace (b) visualization.

the branching arteries and down streams toward the descending aorta as seen in **Figure 10b**. A noticeable vortex appears at the branching point of the IA with the aorta. Two more vortices appear at the bottom section of the aortic arch where the helical flow is generated.

Figure 11 shows flow patterns in the chimney SG case as calculated (a and b) and visualized (c). Large vortices are found at the IA origin and at the SG's intake. Smaller vortices are formed adjacent to the SG.

The flow in the bypass connection with the IA, LCCA and LSA are shown in **Figure 12**. Vortices are found at the exit point from the SG to the IA, at the anastomosis to the LCCA and at the connection point of the bypass with the IA and LSA.

In the hybrid graft case (**Figure 13**), a vortex is seen at the branching point of the graft with the aorta. Smooth flow is seen in the graft and bifurcation. Vortices also appear at the stumps of the IA, LCCA and LSA. Vortices are also found at the bypass connection to the LCCA and LSA (**Figure 14**) and at the LSA stump.

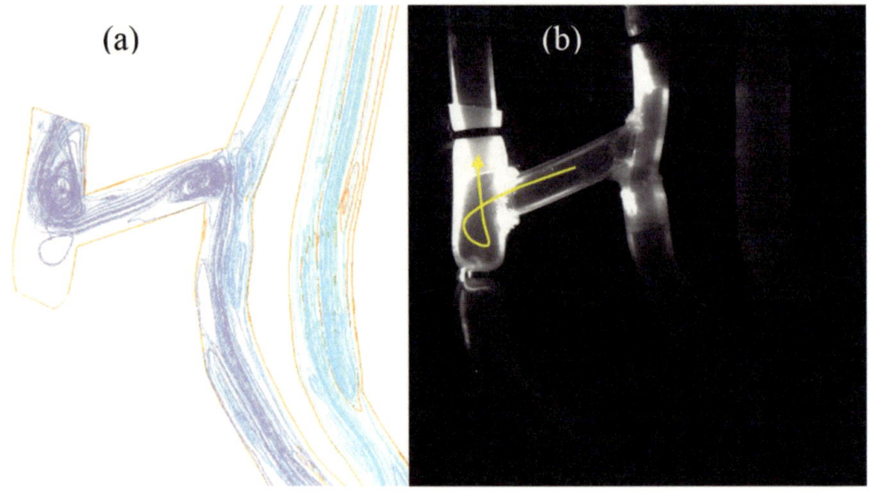

Figure 14. Hybrid bypass (a) CFD particle trace (b) visualization.

4. Discussion

In this study, four numerical models were built and verified using an in vitro experimental method. The models represent aortic arch aneurysm and three different treatment approaches. Comparison of flow patterns between the numerical and experimental results exhibits similar flow regimes in all four models, indicating the validity of the numerical model.

In the aneurysm case, poor hemodynamics is well demonstrated. A large vortex occupies the entire aneurysm sac, and in its center, a single significant stagnation point is observed, especially during diastole as seen in **Figure 9**. This induces poor particle washout and has a high risk of thrombus formation, as shown in previous studies as well [25, 26].

The surgery graft case demonstrated the best hemodynamics performance of all cases. The flow patterns deduced from the numerical analysis are clearly seen in the visualization (**Figures 9–14**). The helical flow that is generated at the aortic arch as seen in the numerical solution is noticed in vitro as well. This type of flow is consistent with findings from literature [27–29].

The chimney case (**Figures 11** and **12**) presented the most disturbed flow of all the three approaches. The large vortex at the insertion point of the stent-graft provokes a strong shear layer and vortical area downstream. A second large vortex at the bend toward the IA is well shown in the numerical model, but was not visually confirmed by the experiments due to local reflections and light scattering from the model. In addition, a series of vortices forming in the stubs of the arteries where they connect to the bypass are clearly seen numerically and experimentally (**Figure 12**).

In the hybrid graft case, a single vortex is noticed at the connection with the aortic arch (seen in **Figure 13**), followed by clean flow in the hybrid grafts branching point. Visualization confirms these findings. The bypass connection between the LSA and LCCA shows a vortex in the stub and is confirmed visually (**Figure 14**). Light did not reach the LCCA, and thus, visional confirmation was not possible.

This study is aimed at validating the numerical models using methods of visualization. The two methods were compared qualitatively by means of flow patterns analysis.

The resulted time-dependent flow presented similar flow regimes and vortex configurations.

The analysis did not take into consideration the motion of the aortic wall [30], and we did not use patient-specific geometries or boundary conditions. Nor turbulence or non-Newtonian effects were considered. Yet, we believe that our models represent the dominant factors influencing the hemodynamics in the different cases.

The reason for model simplifications is that patients' anatomy and physiology come in large variations, and whatever models used will lead to inaccuracy for the global analysis. Therefore, the models are based on representative prototype anatomical geometries, the boundary conditions are based on typical time functions from literature and the flow models were simplified. These assumptions might lead to some inaccuracies in the calculated values for specific patients, especially in WSS and pressure; however, it should not change the overall conclusions of the study.

In conclusion, this study was aimed at introducing a valid numerical model for the different cases. Future research will use more accurate experimental analysis and will examine flow parameters in the different numerical models, including specific regions (like gutter and stumps), wall shear stress, pressure drops and perfusion.

Author details

Asaph Nardi, Barak Even-Chen and Idit Avrahami*

*Address all correspondence to: iditav@ariel.ac.il

Ariel Biomechanics Center, Ariel University, Ariel, Israel

References

[1] Eric M. Isselbacher, *Thoracic and abdominal aortic aneurysms*. Circulation, 2005. 111(6): pp. 816–828.

[2] Eric M. Isselbacher, Epidemiology of thoracic aortic aneurysms, aortic dissection, intramural hematoma, and penetrating atherosclerotic ulcers, in *Aortic Dissection and Related Syndromes*. 2007, Springer US. pp. 3–15.

[3] Knowles, Andrew C., and John D. Kneeshaw. "Aortic dissection." Core Topics in *Cardiac Anesthesia*. 2nd ed. 2012: Cambridge University, UK. (2012): 223.

[4] Al Kindi, A.H., et al., *"Open" approach to aortic arch aneurysm repair*. Journal of the Saudi Heart Association, 2014. 26(3): pp. 152–161.

[5] Ziganshin, B.A. and J.A. Elefteriades, *Deep hypothermic circulatory arrest*. Annals of Cardiothoracic Surgery, 2013. 2(3): pp. 303–315.

[6] Makaroun, M.S., et al., *Five-year results of endovascular treatment with the Gore TAG device compared with open repair of thoracic aortic aneurysms.* Journal of vascular surgery, 2008. 47(5): pp. 912–918.

[7] Moulakakis, K.G., et al., *The chimney-graft technique for preserving supra-aortic branches: a review.* Annals of Cardiothoracic Surgery, 2013. 2(3): pp. 339–346.

[8] Naughton, P.A., et al., *Emergent repair of acute thoracic aortic catastrophes: a comparative analysis.* Archives of Surgery, 2012. 147(3): pp. 243–249.

[9] Avrahami, I., et al., *Hemodynamic and mechanical aspects of fenestrated endografts for treatment of Abdominal Aortic Aneurysm.* European Journal of Mechanics-B/Fluids, 2012. 35: pp. 85–91.

[10] Nardi, A., et al. Hemodynamical Aspects of Endovascular Repair for Aortic Arch Aneurisms. *ASME 2014 12th Biennial Conference on Engineering Systems Design and Analysis*. American Society of Mechanical Engineers, 2014.

[11] Ohrlander, T., et al., The chimney graft: a technique for preserving or rescuing aortic branch vessels in stent-graft sealing zones. *Journal of Endovascular Therapy* 15.4 (2008): 427–432.

[12] Cires, G., et al., *Endovascular debranching of the aortic arch during thoracic endograft repair.* Journal of Vascular Surgery, 2011. 53(6): pp. 1485–1491.

[13] Chuter, T.A.M., et al., *Modular branched stent graft for endovascular repair of aortic arch aneurysm and dissection.* Journal of Vascular Surgery, 2003. 38(4): pp. 859–863.

[14] Brinkman, W.T., W.Y. Szeto, and J.E. Bavaria, *Stent graft treatment for transverse arch and descending thoracic aorta aneurysms.* Current Opinion in Cardiology, 2007. 22(6): p. 510.

[15] Gottardi, R., et al., *An alternative approach in treating an aortic arch aneurysm with an anatomic variant by supraaortic reconstruction and stent-graft placement.* Journal of Vascular Surgery, 2005. 42(2): pp. 357–360.

[16] Ishimaru, S., *Endografting of the aortic arch.* Journal of Endovascular Therapy, 2004. 11(SupplementII): pp. 62–71.

[17] Saleh, H.M. and L. Inglese, *Combined surgical and endovascular treatment of aortic arch aneurysms.* Journal of Vascular Surgery, 2006. 44(3): pp. 460–466. e1.

[18] Yang, J., et al., *Endovascular chimney technique of aortic arch pathologies: a systematic review.* Annals of Vascular Surgery, 2012. 26(7): pp. 1014–1021.

[19] Nardi, A. and I. Avrahami, *Approaches for treatment of aortic arch aneurysm, A numerical study.* Journal of Biomechanics, 2016. BM-D-16-01127.

[20] Brand, M., et al., Clinical, Hemodynamical and Mechanical Aspects of Aortic Aneurisms and Endovascular Repair in Cardiology Research and Clinical Developments. 2013: Nova Publisher, NY.

[21] Buth, J., et al., Combined approach to stent-graft treatment of an aortic arch aneurysm. *Journal of Endovascular Therapy* 5.4 (1998): 329–332.

[22] Yoshida, R., et al., *Total endovascular debranching of the aortic arch.* European Journal of Vascular and Endovascular Surgery, 2011. 42(5): pp. 627–630.

[23] Geisbüsch, P., et al., *Complications after aortic arch hybrid repair.* Journal of Vascular Surgery, 2011. 53(4): pp. 935–941.

[24] Sugiura, K., et al., *The applicability of chimney grafts in the aortic arch.* Journal of Cardiovascular Surgery, 2009. 50(4): pp. 475–481.

[25] Gao, F., A. Qiao, and T. Matsuzawa "Numerical Simulation in Aortic Arch Aneurysm." *Reinhart Grundmann* 12 (2011): 207–222.

[26] Qiao, A., et al. Computational study of stented aortic arch aneurysms. 2005 *IEEE Engineering in Medicine and Biology 27th Annual Conference.* IEEE, 2006.

[27] Hugo, G.B. and H.B. Michael, *Blood flow measurements in the aorta and major arteries with MR velocity mapping.* Journal of Magnetic Resonance Imaging, 1994. 4(2): pp. 119–130.

[28] Morris, L., et al., *3-D numerical simulation of blood flow through models of the human aorta.* Journal of Biomechanical Engineering, 2005. 127: p. 767.

[29] Wen, C.Y., et al., *Investigation of pulsatile flowfield in healthy thoracic aorta models.* Annals of Biomedical Engineering, 2010. 38(2): pp. 391–402.

[30] van Prehn, J., et al., *Toward endografting of the ascending aorta: insight into dynamics using dynamic cine-CTA.* Journal of Endovascular Therapy, 2007. 14(4): pp. 551–560.

Section 4

Thoracic Aortic Aneurysm

Chapter 4

Role of Interventional Treatment of Thoracic Aorta

Ibrahim Akin, Uzair Ansari and
Christoph A. Nienaber

Additional information is available at the end of the chapter

http://dx.doi.org/10.5772/66520

Abstract

An aging western and oriental population coupled with breakthrough advances in modern diagnostic imaging modalities has evoked renewed interest in the hitherto underdiagnosed acute and chronic diseases of the aorta, which also include aortic aneurysm and aortic dissection. Although classical surgical strategies still dominate the clinical management of acute and chronic pathologies of the ascending aorta and the proximal arch region, the emergence of novel endovascular concepts has offered an interesting therapy alternative for the treatment of descending aortic pathology in suitable patients and is highly likely to evolve as the primary treatment strategy in majority of the cases. Moreover, the use of hybrid approaches combining surgical head-vessel debranching and interventional stent-graft implantation in an attempt to improve clinical outcome in aortic arch pathologies has helped avoid the high risk of open arch repair or complete replacement. Notwithstanding these recent advancements, the complex nature of the underlying vascular disease still dictates that the proposed management of every diagnosed patient is discussed in a team constituting cardiologists, cardiac surgeons, anesthesiologists, and radiologists, with the conceptualization of individualized therapeutic strategies and conducted in a center with significant surgical and endovascular experience.

Keywords: aortic dissection, aortic aneurysm, stent graft, endoleak, malperfusion

1. Introduction

The pathophysiological underpinnings initiating the development of thoracic aortic disease are complex and not fully understood. Standard treatment options in most instances have included surgical resection and interposition of vascular prostheses despite the risk of severe complications arising from surgical trauma [1–3]. Although significant advancements in surgical procedures and intraoperative management have mitigated the risk of some of these adverse events, the perioperative mortality and morbidity remains high. Additionally, the changing dynamics of demographic distribution in the western and oriental world have skewed the incidence of disease to an increasingly aging population, a patient group inherently afflicted with a variety of comorbidities, thus foretelling the compounded risk of a sobering surgical outcome.

The use of an endoluminal stent-graft prosthesis initiated as a revolutionary treatment concept more than two decades ago for patients with thoracic aortic disease offered an interesting alternative to open surgery by circumventing certain obvious risks. The induction of reconstructive remodeling of the diseased aorta by triggering a natural healing process through exclusion and depressurization of the aneurysmal process was an innovative interventional approach [4–6], with initial reports suggesting encouraging results for the treatment of various aortic pathologies (e.g., degenerative aneurysm, mycotoxins aneurysm, traumatic injuries, aortic dissections, and penetrating aortic ulcers (PAU)). Scarce randomized data as well as the absence of long-term surveillance of treated patients has strengthened critique against this approach, and with the lack of a satisfying rebuttal, its universal adoption has consequently been hindered [7–10]. This comprehensive chapter describes current indications, techniques, and advancements in endovascular strategies in the treatment of thoracic aortic disease.

2. Classification

Aortic dissection and aortic aneurysm have been listed as the most commonly encountered pathologies of the thoracic aorta. The incidence of aortic dissection in the clinical arena is still relatively rare, with an estimated 2.6–4 cases per 100,000 in the general population reported in a year [11–13]. Statistics reveal that only around 0.5% of the patients presenting with chest or back pain in the emergency room (ER) suffer from aortic dissection [14]. The early phase of this disease, associated with significantly high mortality, is labeled an acute aortic dissection as documented symptom-onset is less than 2 weeks on presentation. Patients surviving the initial 2 weeks without any intervention are classified as suffering from a subacute form, while the chronic patients, who constitute about one-third of all patients with aortic dissection, survive longer than 90 days. The Stanford and DeBakey classifications of aortic dissection are further attempts to group different presentations according to the anatomical location of disease (**Figure 1**). The fundamental distinction lies in the presentation of either a proximal (involving the aortic root or ascending aorta) or distal (beyond the subclavian artery) loci. An untreated proximal aortic dissection is characterized by an initial mortality rate of more than 1% per hour, which if left untreated results in death due to cardiac rupture, tamponade, heart failure from acute aortic regurgitation, or from major coronary closure [11–13]. The prognosis of a distal aortic dissection, popularly known as a Type B aortic dissection, is comparatively better clocking a 30-day mortality rate of about 10% [11–13].

In retrospect, little has been elucidated about the true prevalence and mortality rates of thoracic aortic aneurysms (TAA). An older population-based study reported an age- and gender-adjusted incidence of 5.9 new aneurysms per 100,000 people-year in a Midwestern community over a 30-year period. The median ages for men and women were 65 years and 77 years, respectively, with the primary distribution of cases reflecting an affliction of the ascending aorta in 51% of the patients, of the arch in 11% and of the descending thoracic aorta in 38% [15]. The Crawford classification that attempted to classify these aneurysms based on the origin of distal to the subclavian artery (Types I–IV) has recently been adapted and tweaked by Safi (Type V) [16] (**Figure 2**).

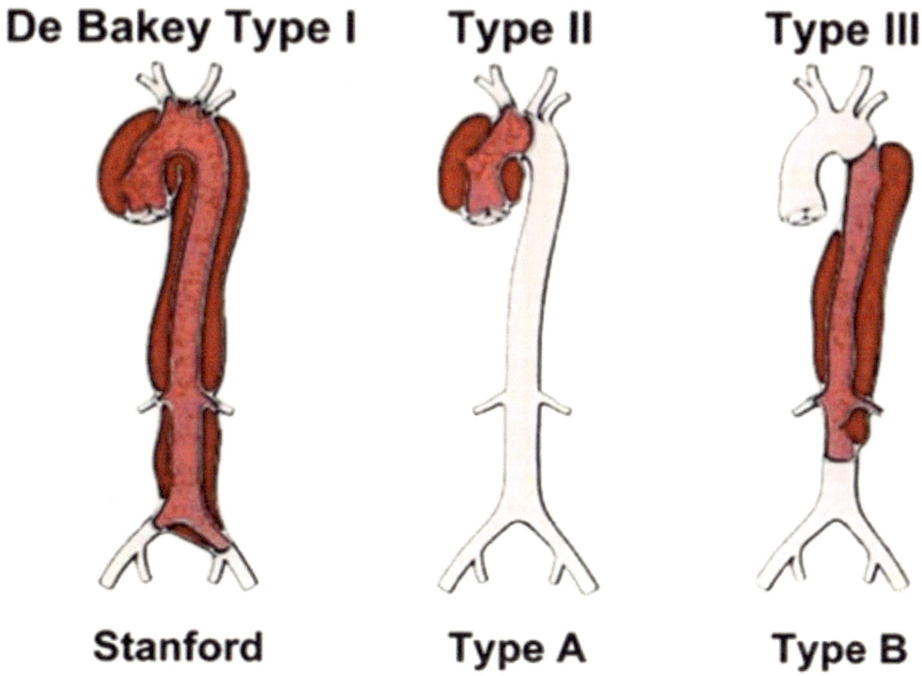

Acuity:

Acute:	<2 weeks after onset
Subacute:	2-8 weeks after onset
Chronic:	>8 weeks after onset

Anatomic location:

Ascending aorta:	Stanford Type A, DeBakey Type II
Ascending and descending aorta:	Stanford Type A, DeBakey Type I
Descending aorta:	Stanford Type B, DeBakey Type III

Pathophysiology:

Class 1: Classical aortic dissection with initimal flap between true and false lumen
Class 2: Aortic intramural hematoma without identifiable intimal flap
Class 3: Intimal tear without hematoma (limited dissection)
Class 4: Atherosclerotic plaque rupture with aortic penetrating ulcer
Class 5: Iatrogenic or traumatic aortic dissection (intra-aortic catherterization, high-speed deceleration injury, blunt chest trauma)

Figure 1. Classification of thoracic aortic dissection.

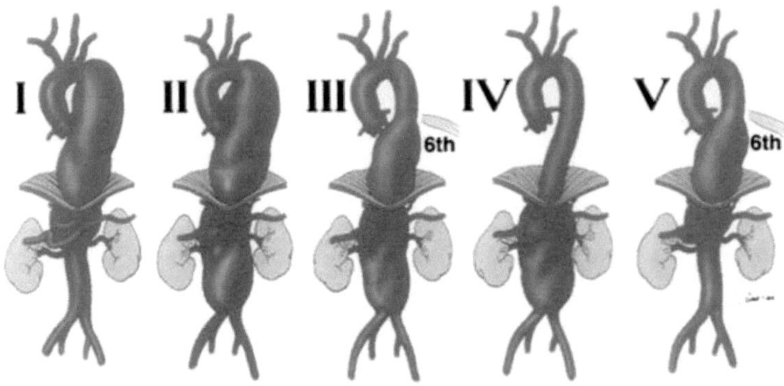

Figure 2. Classification of thoracic aortic aneurysms.

3. Indications for endovascular stent-graft therapy

In the event of an aortic dissection, the sealing of proximal entry tears with a customized stent graft has proven to be the most effective method for excluding a growing aneurysmal false lumen. Although the closure of a distal reentry tear is also desirable, this is not particularly necessary to achieve optimal results [12, 13, 17]. A favorable postinterventional outcome would constitute adequate depressurization and shrinkage of the false lumen, supplemented in an ideal scenario by a complete thrombosis of this lumen with consequent remodeling of the entire dissected aorta [18] (**Figure 3**).

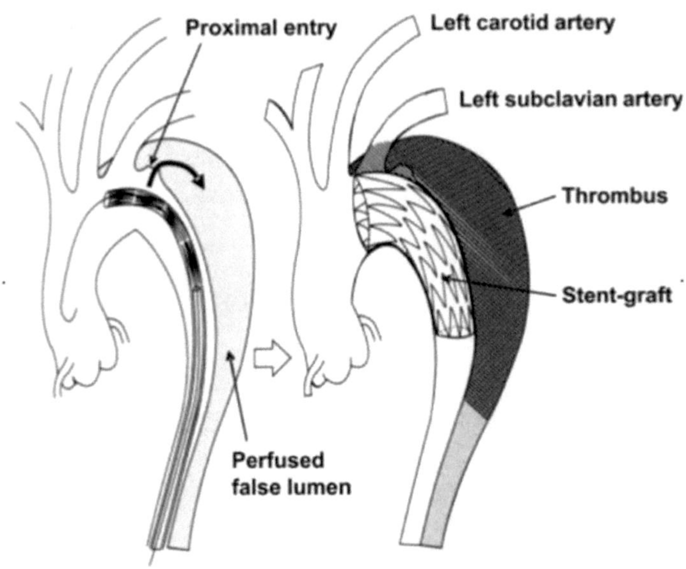

Figure 3. Concept of interventional reconstruction of the dissected aorta with sealing of the proximal entries, depressurization of the false lumen, and initiation of false lumen thrombosis.

Disease etiology
Aortic aneurysms
Atherosclerotic/degenerative
Posttraumatic
Mycotic
Anastomotic
Cystic medial necrosis
Aortitis
Stanford Type B aortic dissection
Acute
Chronic
Giant penetrating ulcer
Traumatic aortic tear
Aortopulmonary fistula
Marfan syndrome
Aneurysm morphology
Aneurysm of the descending aorta
Proximal neck length = 2 cm
<2 cm if supraaortic vessels have been transposed prior stent-graft placement
Distal neck length = 2 cm
Diameter = 6 cm
Patients condition
Preferentially older age
Unfit for open surgical repair or high-risk patients
Chronic obstructive pulmonary disease
Severe coronary heart disease
Severe carotid artery disease
Renal insufficiency
Suitable vascular access site
Life expectancy of more than 6 month

Table 1. Current indication for stent-graft implantation.

The role of percutaneous fenestration in the management of aortic dissection is debatable and should be in all likelihood avoided considering its profile of unproven benefits and interventional risk. The relevance of a team of professionals experienced in treating aortic disease is absolute considering the necessity for a thorough evaluation of the clinical, technical, and anatomical criteria before a treatment strategy has been defined. The general indication for emergency placement of stent grafts has been extended to scenarios where patients have intractable pain associated with a descending dissection, develop a rapidly expanding false lumen diameter, percolate extra-aortic blood (as a sign of imminent rupture), or show signs of a distal malperfusion syndrome [11–13] (**Table 1**). The use of endovascular stent grafting as the primary strategy may be justified in the event of late-onset complications like malperfusion of vital peripheral aortic branches.

4. Anatomical measurements for thoracic aortic pathology

Multi-slice computed tomography (CT) has special relevance in the diagnosis of aortic disease. In addition to the reconstruction of a three-dimensional perspective, certain descriptive features of the thoracic aorta outlining the condition of the aortic wall (atheroma, calcification, and thrombus) as well as shape and size of the aortic pathology (diameter, length, and shape) need to be elucidated before the formulation of treatment strategies [19].

Although an initial CT angiography/magnetic resonance (MR) angiography is considered as the primary diagnostic tool for aortic pathologies, the use of transesophageal echocardiography and intravascular ultrasound to ascertain additional valuable information has also been advised. For instance, flow-sensitive MR sequences or contrast-enhanced TEE not only shows the communication sites between true and false lumen, but it also highlights the dynamic flow pattern in the false lumen prior to stent-graft placement. The use of contrast angiography has limited potential in this scenario as measured values are generally unreliable.

The measurement of vessel diameters is generally not defined by any set of conventional practice and operators usually refer to calculations derived from the inner vessel wall (endothelial trailing edge) hinging their assumption on the basis that this will guarantee some degree of oversizing, a potentially desirable outcome for endograft placement. Our in-house protocol delineates the diameter of the normal appearing proximal aorta (inner edge to edge) measured from a transverse plane perpendicular to the long axis of the aorta (preferentially from contrast-enhanced multi-slice CT images) (**Figure 4**).

The evaluation of access vessels for size and tortuosity is also pertinent because stent-graft delivery systems are quite large (up to 24F), and there is an associated risk of significant trauma to the femoral access site and iliac arteries. Severe aortic angulation or tortuosity, friable atheroma or thrombus lining the aortic wall, and aortic pathology involving the ascending aorta are some features that preclude the use of thoracic stent grafts. Additionally, the role of appropriate peri-interventional image reconstruction in aortic arch pathology is further cemented when considering the placement of a stent graft for a Type B dissection, where the demarcation of nearby aortic branches (including the left subclavian or left common carotid artery) is vital.

http://dx.doi.org/10.5772/66520

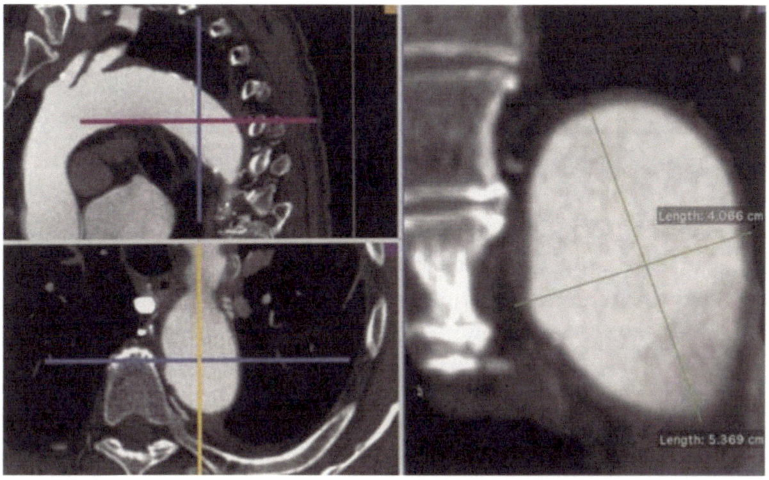

Figure 4. CT scan of a patient with dilated thoracic aorta. Due to the fact that the aorta follows a curved and three-dimensionally tortuous path, the axial scans are inadequate for measuring aortic diameters, as are sagittal and coronal planes for measuring aortic lengths.

5. Initial treatment

An acute aortic disease is a medical emergency and suspected patients require urgent admission to an intensive care or monitoring unit with an emphasis on immediate diagnostic evaluation [20]. Initial management strategies include the treatment of pain and maintenance of a systolic blood pressure of 110 mmHg with the use of morphine sulphate and intravenous beta-blockers (metoprolol, esmolol, or labetolol), respectively. The use of additional anti-hypertensives like angiotensin-converting enzyme inhibitors or vasodilators like sodium nitroprusside has been prescribed in refractory cases, while the intravenous use of verapamil or diltiazem is recommended for patients in whom beta-blockers are contraindicated. Although monotherapy with beta-blockers sufficiently controls cases of mild hypertension, the addition of sodium nitroprusside at an initial dose of 0.3 μg/kg/min proves to be an effective combination in a severe hypertensive state. A careful evaluation for blood loss, pericardial effusion, or heart failure (by echocardiography) is a prerequisite before administering volume in normotensive or hypotensive patients. Additionally, the control of heart rate is of utmost importance in this scenario [21]. Hemodynamic instability compounds to the gravity of the clinical situation, with patients often requiring endotracheal intubation, mechanical ventilation, and urgent bedside transesophageal echocardiography or rapid CT for confirmation of the provisional diagnosis. In rare instances, the diagnosis of cardiac tamponade as quantified by transthoracic echocardiography may justify an immediate sternotomy in order to obtain surgical access to the ascending aorta, thus reducing the risk of shock, ischemic brain damage, and circulatory arrest.

6. Technique of endovascular stent-graft placement

The use of individually selected stent grafts to cover up to 20 cm (and sometimes even more) of the diseased aorta relies on measurements derived from different diagnostic modalities. These tests also have certain additional benefits. The transesophageal echocardiography is mandatory for detection of small entries, while contrast-enhanced CT (Computed tomography) angiograms have proven to be the preferred tool for diagnosis of unstable patients in an emergency situation. The use of intravascular ultrasound (IVUS), using a 10 MHz ultrasound catheter-mounted transducer with the potential of manual maneuverability through the diseased aorta, can be used to better identify communications, partial thrombosis, or other anomalies.

The operative placement of an endovascular stent graft is usually performed in a Cathlab or a hybrid operating room equipped with digital angiography and necessary support for general anesthesia (a compulsory prerequisite for all patients). The femoral artery generally serves as the access-site as it could typically accommodate a 20–24 stent-graft system. After the employment of the Seldinger technique to position the initial sheath, a 260 cm stiff wire (e.g., Amplatzer) is placed over a pigtail catheter and navigated along with a soft wire in the true lumen under both fluoroscopic and transesophageal ultrasound guidance. The "embracement technique" augmented by the use of two pigtail catheters could prove useful in maintaining the true lumen during complex cases when multiple reentries into the abdominal aorta are required. Essentially, a catheter inserted via the left brachial artery navigates through the true aortic lumen and meets the femoral pigtail catheter in the true lumen of the abdominal aorta, thence pulling it up into the aortic arch. This technique ensures the definitive positioning of the stiff guide wire within the true lumen necessary for the ensuing endovascular intervention. The subsequent launch of the stent graft is performed by carefully advancing the graft over the stiff wire in the true lumen while briefly maintaining a low blood pressure through rapid right ventricular pacing [22]. To improve apposition of the stent struts to the aortic wall in the event of incomplete sealing of the proximal thoracic communications, a latex balloon may be shortly inflated at the target site postdeployment of graft and sealing of entry flap. Doppler-ultrasound and contrast fluoroscopy are useful techniques instrumental in confirming the immediate result and play a vital role when initiating adjunctive maneuvers. The navigation of wires and instruments is less cumbersome in the setting of a thoracic aortic aneurysm (TAA) or aortic ulcer; however, meticulous intraprocedural ultrasound imaging and fluoroscopy are essential to monitor the interventional progress. The close vicinity of the left subclavian artery origin to the primary tear in Type B dissections presents a unique anatomical problem, often requiring a radical solution. A complete closure of the left subclavian artery (LSA) ostium may be necessary at times to ensure the proper placement and debranching of the stent graft, else use of extra-anatomical bypasses would have to be considered [23]. Observational evidence dictates that prophylactic surgical maneuvers are not always required but could be performed electively after the endovascular intervention in the event of developing ischemia. Additionally, the existence of potential supra-aortic variants (e.g., presence of a lusorian artery, an incomplete vertebra-basilar system, or vertebral arteries directly originating from the arch) must be considered before the intentional occlusion of LSA [24].

7. Device sizing and length

A key factor influencing strategies in aortic dissection and TAA interventions is the length of the true lumen that needs scaffolding with an endoprosthesis. The instinctual choice between covering primarily the proximal entry point and alternatively lining a longer length of the true lumen (where the descending thoracic aorta down to the level of the diaphragm is also treated) can significantly alter the course and prognosis of the intervention. Although a longer scaffold provides potentially greater stability and is associated with lower recurrence, the grave risk of potential paraplegia resulting from compromise in spinal arterial supply serves as the single biggest reason to avoid extensive coverage. Observational evidence indicates that stent-graft coverage exceeding 20 cm, previous abdominal aortic surgery, overstenting of the LSA, or use of the left mammary artery for coronary bypass is associated with an increased risk of spinal ischemia. Essentially, all scenarios leading to compromised collateral flow in the spinal cord arterial network are associated with an increased risk for neurological complications, thus underlining the need to avoid overstenting the LSA or use long stent grafts. The angiographic identification of the anterior spinal artery in this scenario has recently shown prognostic relevance.

The disadvantage of shorter coverage lengths is primarily associated with potential multiple reentries presenting themselves in the distal portions of the descending aorta and maintaining perfusion of the false lumen despite proximal entry-site closure. This deviant presentation can be managed by the use of uncovered bare metal stents ensuring distal reapposition of the dissecting lamella without any compromise to abdominal side branches or spinal arteries, in effect sustaining the distal extension of the scaffolding concept of endoluminal repair.

The proximal aspect of the device should be sized to the internal luminal diameter of the aorta, close to the left subclavian origin in order to achieve attachment and fixation at the proximal "neck." TAA interventions may require a degree of device oversizing by about 10–15%, while the endoprosthesis used in aortic dissection should never be oversized. Fatal complications are associated with excessive device oversizing, typically as a result of ensuing trauma to the aortic wall, thus resulting in either a retrograde dissection into the arch or conversion of a Type B dissection into a Type A dissection. Cases of aortic perforation and formation of pseudoaneurysms have also been reported in literature. The countereffects of oversizing further distally into the descending thoracic aorta include the risk of tears in the membrane between the two channels, thus forming a new reentry point, and consequently sustaining the ongoing pressurized perfusion of the false lumen. However, if absolute measures do dictate the extensive scaffolding of the aortic lumen, the operator could choose to use two different shorter grafts instead of a single long graft. The final decision represents a compromise between the reduced number of modular junctions and additional frictional forces associated with the deployment of a long stent graft. The concurrent employment of two stent grafts, when deemed necessary, requires them being fashioned in a "telescopic" manner, with the amount of overlap exceeding 30 mm in straight anatomic segments and measuring up to 50 mm or more in the angulated or curved segments of the aorta. The geometry of the presumed junction between the grafts provides some assistance in estimating the length of overlap required at the connecting zones. A key deciding factor in this situation is the length of the radius of the curve, with shorter radii requiring a longer stent overlap on the lesser curve. Another prominent factor influencing the decision regarding overlap is the degree of support provided by the native aorta at the modular junction. If the junction occurs in the sac of a large fusiforme aneurysm rather than in a segment of aorta with a normal diameter, the required overlap should be longer. The reason for this approach is a tendency for the graft to move out toward the greater curve of the aneurysmatic aortic segment due to mechanical forces associated with the pulsatile motion of the aorta, potentially causing a migration or a disconnection of the modular components.

8. Extended scaffolding with bare stents

The general consensus on management of entry tears dictates treatment with a covered stent graft, while the remaining distal thoracic or even abdominal aorta may be additionally supported by uncovered stents [25]. In selecting the suitable stent graft, the following principles should be followed:

- An appropriate size and diameter is crucial to avoid erosion through the aortic wall and to assure optimal conformability.
- The flexibility of the endoprosthesis and its release with a deployment mechanism should permit ease of use and provide accurate placement at the desired zone.
- The fragility of the dissected wall directs the use of a stent graft that is not dependent on balloon expansion for deployment or postdeployment modeling. Our experience suggests that the use of a self-expanding endoprosthesis with a nitinol-based architecture using limited radial force (in case of aortic dissection) is helpful in avoiding any untoward ballooning.

9. Landing zone

The three-dimensional mechanical forces associated with the pulsatile flow that "play" on an endoprosthesis in the thoracic aorta are far greater and more complex than those in the abdominal aorta. It is for this reason that an extremely stable graft-anchorage and optimal graft-apposition are prerequisites for a satisfying result. The proximal and distal landing zones should ideally be free of aortic wall atheroma or thrombi and circumscribe 15 mm in length. The contemporary hypothesis suggesting that the left subclavian artery is a natural barrier beyond which it is impossible to deploy stent grafts has been now rendered redundant.

The suitable presentation of the aortic arch between the left subclavian artery and the origin of the left common carotid artery, coupled with its relatively horizontal orientation in comparison to the aorta distal to the LSA, has encouraged interventionists to use this segment

http://dx.doi.org/10.5772/66520

of the aorta as a preferred anchor zone (with or without bypassing the LSA). To ascertain optimal cerebral circulation, it is considered prudent to perform a preinterventional digital subtraction angiography (DSA), CT, or magnetic resonance angiography. This could help identify patients with an incomplete circle of Willis or other limitations or abnormalities of cerebral vascular supply. In patients affected with a cerebrovascular pathology, prophylactic measures such as carotid-subclavian bypass might be considered prior to the stent-associated covering of the LSA. An obvious alternative is the use of bare stents proximally for better alignment while foregoing the risk of occluding a vital branch.

10. Hybrid arch procedures

The relative proximity of supra-aortic branches needing preservation poses a strict interventional challenge, considering that the aortic arch anatomy and pathology is complicated by varying degrees of length and angulation [26–28]. The traditional open arch surgical reconstruction techniques requiring perioperative hypothermic cardiac arrest, extracorporeal circulation, and selective cerebral perfusion have been shown to manage aortic arch pathologies effectively. However, these major surgical procedures carry the risk of significant mortality, paraplegia, and cerebral stroke. Younger patients with a smaller risk-profile qualify for such an open repair, while high-risk patients constitute the group of candidates ill-suited for this surgical approach. Hybrid arch procedures are a combination of methods preserving cerebral perfusion (like the debranching bypass with supra-aortic vessel transposition) on the one hand, while objectively providing patient-centric solutions for complex aortic arch lesions through thoracic endografting on the other (**Figure 5**). Hybrid arch procedures are performed without hypothermic circulatory arrest or extracorporeal circulation, thus expanding the treatable population demographic to older and high-risk patients with severe comorbidities currently not eligible for open surgical repair.

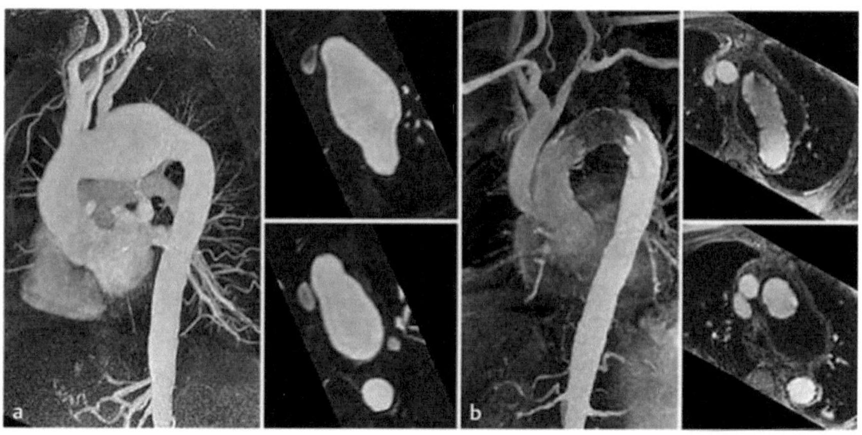

Figure 5. Contrast-medium enhanced MR-angiography of the aorta in a case of an arch aneurysm. (a) Aneurysm of the aortic arch involving the supra-aortic branches. (b) Result after hybrid procedure with debranching of the supraaortic vessels and stent-graft placement in the aortic arch.

11. Aftercare and long-term follow-up

The long-term care of patients successfully treated for an acute aortic dissection is pivoted on the appreciation of this disease as a systemic illness. Estimates suggest that nearly one-third of patients surviving an acute dissection of the thoracic aorta will either experience complications like extension of the dissection and late aortic rupture or require surgical correction of a newly formed aortic aneurysm, within 5 years of initial presentation [29]. All patients merit aggressive medical therapy, follow-up visits, and serial CT-imaging. The medical management of these patients is primarily centered on therapy with beta-blockers, in essence serving as the cornerstone of successful aftercare. High blood pressure values and steeper curves representing changes in the blood volume and pressure (dp/dt) have been shown to accelerate aortic expansion in Marfan's syndrome and also in patients with chronic abdominal aortic aneurysms (AAA). The aim in patients with thoracic aortic disease is to balance blood pressure values to less than 135/80 mmHg, while patients diagnosed with Marfan's syndrome are advised to maintain blood pressure levels below 130/80 mmHg [11–13]. Additionally, an adequate control of heart rate under 60 beats per minute has been associated with significantly fewer secondary adverse events (aortic expansion, recurrent aortic dissection, aortic rupture, and/or need for aortic surgery) in Type B aortic dissection patients [21].

Serial CT imaging of the aorta is an essential component of long-term management (before and after surgery or stent-graft placement). The choice of imaging modality, CT or magnetic resonance, is dependent on institutional availability and expertise. Past recommendations have suggested follow-up imaging at 1-, 3-, 6-, 9-, and 12-month intervals following discharge, and annually thereafter [11–13]. This aggressive strategy, in effect, underlines the observation that both hypertension and aortic expansion/dissection are common and not easily predicted in the first months following hospital discharge. The risk of dissection progression and aneurysm formation anywhere along the entire length of the aorta cements the need for consistent follow-up imaging of the complete thoracic aorta and in exceptional cases, imaging of the thoracoabdominal as well as abdominal aorta.

12. Management of complications

12.1. Endoleaks

An endoleak is a condition defined by the persistence of blood flow outside the endovascular stent-graft lumen, contained within the aneurysm sac, or in certain cases adjacent to the vascular segment treated by the stent graft. Endoleaks generally persist for a long duration, with a few eventually developing a late aneurysmal rupture, while some may also resolve and close spontaneously.

The classification of endoleaks according to time of onset permits their grouping into "primary endoleaks," when it occurs during the perioperative period (lesser than 30 days) or secondary leak when it is detected later. Further subcategorization requires precise information on periprosthetic blood flow. A Type I endoleak is an indicator of a persistent perigraft

http://dx.doi.org/10.5772/66520

channel of blood flow caused by an inadequate seal at either the proximal (I-a) or distal (I-b) stent-graft end or attachment zones. A Type II endoleak is attributed to retrograde flow into the aneurysmal sac via aortic side branches, while a Type III endoleak is caused by component disconnection (III-a) or fabric tear, fabric disruption, or graft disintegration (III-b). Type III-b can be further stratified as minor (<2 mm), or major (>2 mm). The Type IV endoleak is caused by blood flow through an intact but otherwise porous fabric, observed during the first 30 days after stent-graft implantation. If an endoleak is detected on imaging studies but the precise source cannot be determined, the endoleak is categorized as an endoleak of undefined origin.

Various strategies have been outlined for the treatment of endoleaks. The conservative line of management, essentially constituting strict observation and follow-up is especially suggested for Type II and Type IV endoleaks. An endovascular reintervention (e.g., balloon-inflation and/or implantation of an additional stent graft) is suggested for the management of Type I and Type III endoleaks. If these endovascular maneuvers fail in their attempt to exclude the aneurysm from circulation, the resulting increase in TAA-diameters could be corrected by open surgery.

13. Aneurysm evolution after stent-graft treatment

The thoracic aorta is defined by a set of unique anatomical features and habits a distinctive biomechanical and hemodynamic environment, which explains some of the rare late complications specific to device use seen in this region. The descending thoracic aorta, unlike the abdominal aorta, is relatively mobile in the thorax and is subject to complex and vigorous three-dimensional motion. The only points of fixation are the aortic root and sites of origin of major branches, thereby permitting the mobility of a long aortic segment extending from the LSA to the celiac artery. This contributes to the elongation, angulation, and eventual enlargement of the thoracic aorta between these points, thus promoting the development of an aneurysm. The mechanical forces exert a complex pattern of dynamic circumferential, radial, and axial forces on thoracic stent grafts, resulting in a stress field significantly different than that exerted on abdominal stent grafts. It is, however, still relatively rare to see aneurysms develop in the dissected aorta post stent-graft treatment. The relevance of strict clinical and imaging follow-up to monitor anatomical changes in the thoracic aorta is highlighted by the fact that the development of a false lumen thrombosis secondary to thoracic endografting is essential to the prevention of late aortic expansion.

A pertinent issue of concern is the fate of the distal aortic segment despite successful thoracic stent-graft placement. In the presence of large reentry points, the thoracoabdominal segment of the false lumen has a tendency to remain patent and remodel completely, setting the stage for late complications such as aneurysmal enlargement at the proximal or distal end of the stent graft. Some other complications include perforations of the fragile aortic intima by the ends of the metallic stent (especially in the early phase of acute aortic dissection), and injuries caused by stiff guide-wires and device manipulation potentially setting the stage for an evolving aneurysm. The risk of these complications is noticeably diminished by the introduction of a more flexible and soft tip delivery system aided by minimally traumatic thoracic guide-wires specifically designed for these interventions. Additionally, the time required to perform an endovascular intervention could provide insight to complications such as stroke or bleeding; both of which could be significantly reduced by experienced interventionists requiring less than 30 min to complete a case. It has been also suggested that the patency of the abdominal aortic false lumen may be related to persisting communications between the true and false lumen. Treatment of these communications at the level of distal thoracic and abdominal aorta could potentially obliterate the false lumen and reduce the aortic diameter. In clinical practice, however, the closure is difficult to achieve because of the proximity or involvement of the visceral branches. Another late complication of graft treatment is related to the mechanical weakness of dissected aortic walls causing distention of the aorta beyond the portion covered by the stent graft. Prevention of these complications can be partially achieved during the primary procedure by ensuring adequate landing zones proximal and distal to the stent graft, and closure of large fenestrations along the length of the false lumen. The use of a provisional bare metal stent as a distal extension to the stent graft has been reported to facilitate aortic remodeling and help completely repair the distal dissected segments without compromising important side-branches (Provisional Extension To Induce Complete Attachement after stent-graft implantation (PETTICOAT) technique) [25]. This would address the problem of persistent perfusion within the false lumen as well as any increase in aneurysmal size.

14. Stent-graft infection

The infected prosthetic graft represents a rare complication that could be difficult to diagnose despite extensive work up, with consensus reached only after thorough analysis of imaging, hematological, and clinical parameters. The presence of air, soft tissue accumulation, and progressive enlargement of the aneurysm sac is usually pathognomonic, and suspicious changes spotted in imaging coupled with raised markers of systemic inflammation and clinical symptoms are generally suggestive of an infective process. The diagnostic use of positron emission tomography (PET) radionuclide studies is a helpful tool in most cases. Prior to initiation of treatment against thoracic endograft infections, data concerning diagnostic certainty, pathogenesis of the infecting microbe, the extent of infection, the presenting features, and the medical co-morbidities of a given patient need to be evaluated.

As with the treatment of all prosthetic graft infections, multiple management strategies have been proposed in this scenario. These include a conservative line of treatment with targeted intravenous antibiotics or also alternatively by direct puncture and application into the peri-graft space; insertion of another stent graft into the potentially infected graft or excision of the infected stent graft with debridement of the surrounding tissue; and in-situ/extra-anatomic vascular reconstruction. Irrespective of the applied strategy, the treatment of aortic graft infection remains difficult and problematic. In the absence of management algorithms defining treatment strategies in the varying forms of presentation and degrees of infection, individualized therapies need to be devised while weighing the risks in each scenario. In general, a decision must be made as to whether treatment is to be potentially curative or palliative. The curative treatment approach encompasses an aggressive open surgery, justified only in certain cases in lieu of the relatively high mortality associated with the procedure.

The palliative approach suggests placement of an endovascular graft (graft-in-graft approach) thereby preventing the risk of life-threatening bleeding or fistulation. Patients with complex graft disease should always be treated in experienced centers equipped to conduct all treatment variations.

15. Retrograde Type A dissection following stent-graft placement

There have been cases reporting a proximal aortic dissection after placement of an endograft; the incidence of this complication, according to existing data, ranges presumably between 1 and 2% and generally occurs shortly after the intervention [30, 31]. Chest pain or symptoms of an ischemic heart or brain should immediately alert the suspicion that a Type B dissection has modified itself to a Type A dissection, with a higher morbidity and mortality risk. An emergency Computed tomography angiography (CTA) and subsequent surgery are the only lifesaving options for the patient. There are several reasons why Type A dissections may occur after stent-graft placement in the descending thoracic aorta (**Table 2**).

The initial misinterpretation of a Type A dissection as a Type B dissection
Spread of the dissection into the ascending aorta or aortic arch due improper placement of the stent graft relatively distant to the LSA, or the possible maneuvering into the false lumen
Under- or oversizing of the stent graft, with consequent leaks or additional injuries to the aortic wall
Malapposition of the stent graft to the aortic wall at the proximal landing zone resulting in subsequent collapse of the proximal stent graft
Ballooning of the proximal end of the stent graft resulting in injury of the diseased aortic wall, thus causing the extension of the dissection in the aortic arch and ascending aorta
Development of a Type A dissection independent of the existing Type B dissection

Table 2. Cause of Type A aortic dissection after stent-graft implantation.

In these cases, it is of absolute importance to advance the guide-wire, catheter, and endograft in the true lumen only. If doubts persist concerning the correct positioning of the guide wire (in the true or false lumen), the use of angiography and transoesophageal echocardiography is instrumental before initiation of the next step. Signs differentiating the true from the false lumen include luminal size, where the false aortic lumen is usually larger than the true lumen, as well as flow at entry, which is generally directed into the false lumen. This explains the damping of the pulse amplitude and a poorly palpable pulse in many of these patients.

Precise measurement of the proximal aortic dimensions is essential for the selection of the size of stent graft and successful sealing of aortic tears. In Type B dissection, the stent graft is normally placed with its proximal end directly at the origin of the LSA. The proximal landing of a stent graft is usually close to the LSA, even though the tear could be in the middle portion; so performed, when considering the possibility of a dissection membrane developing a new tear between LSA and proximal end of the stent graft. In successful cases, angiography demonstrates a good result with complete sealing of the leak and absence of signs showing renewed opacification of the false lumen. Occasionally, a stiff endograft chafes on the fragile dissection membrane and a new endoleak may develop. This could possibly require additional stent grafting or eventually lead to open surgery.

16. Paraplegia after stent-graft placement

The risk of spinal cord ischemia is of significant concern post stent-graft placement as there is a frequent need to cover multiple intercostal arteries as also the artery of Adamkiewitz (the single prominent intersegmental branch from the aorta at the lower thoracic or upper lumbar level). Interestingly, around 3–12% of the stent-graft patients treated for aneurysms, dissections, ulcers, intramural hematoma, or aortic traumatic transsection are at risk to develop spinal cord ischemia. Although occlusion of important radicular arteries that originate from vertebral, intercostal, and lumbar arteries is primarily responsible for ischemia of the spinal cord, associated factors such as ischemia-reperfusion and hypotension may also play a causal role in the development of paraplegia. This is a telling contradiction to the widely held impression that the coverage of the segmental artery or the orifices of the intercostal/interlumbar arteries by the stent graft represents the single possible and most critical cause of spinal ischemia. Measures to prevent occurrence of paraplegia in stent-graft patients should include several aspects (**Table 3**).

Screening for high-risk patients
o Age > 75
o Anticipated endograft coverage between T9 and T12 (location of anterior spinal artery)
o Coverage of long segment (>20 cm)
o Compromised collateral pathways (e.g., LIMA as coronary artery bypass, infrarenal surgical aortic repair)
o Long extent of atherosclerotic lesions
-Early detection of spinal cord ischemia
o Somatosensory-evoked potentials
o Motor-evoked potentials
-Monitoring of cerebral or spinal cord perfusion and drainage (spinal tap decreases intrathecal pressure to 10–15 cm H_2O to generate space for collateral arteries to fill and perfuse better)
-Prevention of perioperative hypotension

Table 3. Factors influencing the rate of paraplegia.

Symptoms of paraplegia or paraparesis could be possibly reversed if a spinal tap is introduced without any delay and arterial perfusion pressure is maintained at a systolic pressure of 140 mmHg by pharmacological means or volume replenishment.

http://dx.doi.org/10.5772/66520

17. Stroke after stent-graft placement

Stroke is a grave complication occurring post stent-graft replacement and reports of incidence vary between 0 and 18%. The instrumentation in the aortic arch has been known to produce an embolic shower in the brain, and the use of guidewires and catheters as well as bulky delivery systems carrying the stent grafts in endovascular interventions in this region supplements to the risk. The need for balloon dilatation of stent grafts adds to the possibility of dislodgement of particles from the aortic arch. It is also well known that proper flushing of the stent-graft delivery system does not guarantee the elimination of air contained in the crimped stent graft. Moreover, bubbles are also released with the deployment of the stent graft. The confirmation of an open contralateral vertebral artery with correct formation of the basilar trunk and absence of intracranial branch anomalies is a basic prerequisite in patients in whom subclavian artery closure is considered.

In summary, there is an absolute need to completely define the left vertebral artery with depiction of its origin, patency, and size, as well as the size and condition of the right vertebral artery including the constitution of the basilar artery and its branches before conducting a procedure involving the closure of the LSA. In patients with compromised cerebral circulation, prior diagnosis of the four vessels with cerebral angiography is the recommended standard. When the left vertebral artery takes off from the aortic arch, occlusion of the LSA can result in severe ischemia of the left arm. If the left vertebral artery takes off from an aneurysm that is being excluded, it could result in a Type II endoleak, a severe steal phenomenon or even present as an ipsilateral posterior stroke. In such cases, a transposition of the LSA prior to the intervention is required.

18. Conclusions

Endovascular stent grafting represents an exciting therapeutic advancement and has emerged as an alternative therapy to open surgical repair in thoracic aortic pathologies. Although it is apparent that high-risk patients will benefit from this technology, the exact role of stent grafting needs to be defined as long-term data is constantly accumulated and analyzed, and further influenced by evolving devices and technology. Rather than replacing conventional surgical treatment, endovascular repair will likely play a complementary role and offer a less invasive option in the treatment armamentarium. Clearly, there are limitations to both approaches; however, while high-risk surgery is defined by clinical parameters, comorbidities and physiological reserve, contraindications for endovascular stent-graft treatment are defined mostly by anatomical criteria such as a too wide aorta to provide landing zones for an endoprosthesis or already irreversible paraplegia. Nevertheless, treatment should be carried out only in a center with experience in both endovascular and surgical procedures, and with adequate technical facilities. Treatment of thoracic aortic pathologies should be subject to prior multidisciplinary discussion, particularly with regard to risks of conversion and need for cardiopulmonary bypass. All patients should have access to a structural follow-up plan offering both regular clinical assessment and professional imaging follow-up by CT or MR angiography.

Conflict of interest

No conflict of interest for authors.

Author details

Ibrahim Akin[1*], Uzair Ansari[1] and Christoph A. Nienaber[2]

*Address all correspondence to: ibrahim.akin@umm.de

1 Universitätsmedizin Mannheim, Mannheim, Germany

2 Royal Brompton Hospital and Harefield Trust, London, UK

References

[1] Cooley DA, DeBakey ME. Resection of the thoracic aorta with replacement by homograft for aneurysms and constrictive lesions. J Thorac Surg 1955; 29: 66–100.

[2] Svensson LG, Crawford ES, Hess KR, Coselli JS, Safi HJ. Experience with 1,509 patients undergoing thoracoabdominal aortic operations. J Vasc Surg 1993; 17: 357–368.

[3] Trimarchi S, Nienaber CA, Rampoldi V, Myrmel T, Suzuki T, Bossone E, Tolva V, Deeb MG, Upchurch GR Jr, Cooper JV, Fang J, Isselbacher EM, Sundt TM 3rd, Eagle KA; IRAD Investigators. Role and results of surgery in acute type B aortic dissection: insight from the International Registry of Aortic Dissection (IRAD). Circulation 2006; 114(1 Suppl): I357–I364.

[4] Volodos NL, Shekhanin VE, Karpovich IP, Troian VI, Gur'ev IuA. A self-fixing synthetic blood vessel endoprosthesis. Vestn Khir Im I I Grek 1986; 137: 123–125.

[5] Dake MD, Miller DC, Semba CP, Mitchell RS, Walker PJ, Liddell RP. Transluminal placement of endovascular stent-grafts for the treatment of descending thoracic aortic aneurysms. N Engl J Med 1994; 331: 1729–1734.

[6] Nienaber CA, Fattori R, Lund G, Dieckmann C, Wolf W, von Kodolitsch Y, Nicolas V, Pierangeli A. Nonsurgical reconstruction of thoracic aortic dissection by stent-graft placement. N Engl J Med 1999; 340: 1539–1545.

[7] Coady MA, Rizzo JA, Hammond GL, Pierce JG, Kopf GS, Elefteriades JA. Penetrating ulcer of the thoracic aorta: what is it? How do we recognize it? How do we manage it?. J Vasc Surg 1998; 27: 1006–1015.

[8] Evangelista A, Mukherjee D, Mehta RH, O'Gara PT, Fattori R, Cooper JV, Smith DE, Oh JK, Hutchison S, Sechtem U, Isselbacher EM, Nienaber CA, Pape LA, Eagle KA; International Registry of Aortic Dissection (IRAD) Investigators. Acute intramural hematoma of the aorta: a mystery in evolution. Circulation 2006; 111: 1063–1070.

[9] Ganaha F, Miller DC, Sugimoto K, Do YS, Minamiguchi H, Saito H, Mitchell RS, Dake MD. Prognosis of aortic intramural hematoma with and without penetrating atherosclerotic ulcer: a clinical and radiological analysis. Circulation 2002; 106: 342–348.

[10] Nienaber CA, von Kodolitsch Y, Petersen B, Loose R, Helmchen U, Haverich A, Spielmann RP. Intramural hemorrhage of the thoracic aorta. Diagnostic and therapeutic implications. Circulation 1995; 92: 1465–1472.

[11] Erbel R, Alfonso F, Boileau C, Dirsch O, Eber B, Haverich A, Rakowski H, Struyven J, Radegran K, Sechtem U, Taylor J, Zolikofer C, Klein WW, Mulder B, Providencia LA; Task Force on Aortic Dissection, European Society of Cardiology. Diagnosis and management of aortic dissection. Eur Heart J 2001; 22: 1642–1681.

[12] Svensson LG, Kouchoukos NT, Miller DC, Bavaria JE, Coselli JS, Curi MA, Eggebrecht H, Elefteriades JA, Erbel R, Gleason TG, Lytle BW, Mitchell RS, Nienaber CA, Roselli EE, Safi HJ, Shemin RJ, Sicard GA, Sundt TM 3rd, Szeto WY, Wheatley GH 3rd; Society of Thoracic Surgeons Endovascular Surgery Task Force. Expert consensus document on the treatment of descending thoracic disease using endovascular stent-grafts. Ann Thorac Surg 2008; 85(1 Suppl): S1–S41.

[13] Hagan PG, Nienaber CA, Isselbacher EM, Bruckman D, Karavite DJ, Russman PL, Evangelista A, Fattori R, Suzuki T, Oh JK, Moore AG, Alouf JF, Pape LA, Gaca C, Sechtem U, Lenferink S, Deutsch HJ, Diedrichs H, Marcos y Robles J, Llovet A, Gilon D, Das SK, Armstrong WF, Deeb GM, Eagle KA. The International Registry of Acute Aortic Dissection (IRAD): new insights into an old disease. JAMA 2000; 283: 897–903.

[14] Kodolitsch Y, Schwarz AG, Nienaber CA. Clinical prediction of acute aortic dissection. Arch Intern Med 2000; 160: 2977–2982.

[15] Clouse WD, Hallett JW Jr, Schaff HV, Gayari MM, Ilstrup DM, Melton LJ 3rd. Improved prognosis of thoracic aneurysms: a population-based study. JAMA 1998; 280: 1926–1929.

[16] Crawford ES, Crawford JL, Safi HJ, Coselli JS, Hess KR, Brooks B, Norton HJ, Glaeser DH. Thoracoabdominal aortic aneurysms: preoperative and intraoperative factors determining immediate and long-term results of operations in 605 patients. J Vasc Surg 1986; 3: 389–404.

[17] Swee W, Dake MD. Endovascular management of thoracic dissection. Circulation 2009; 117: 1460–1473.

[18] Tsai TT, Evangelista A, Nienaber CA, Myrmel T, Meinhardt G, Cooper JV, Smith DE, Suzuki T, Fattori R, Llovet A, Froehlich J, Hutchison S, Distane A, Sundt T, Beckman J, Januzzi JL Jr, Isselbacher EM, Eagle KA; International Registry of Acute Aortic Dissection. Partial thrombosis of the false lumen in patients with acute type B aortic dissection. N Engl J Med 2007; 357: 349–359.

[19] Salvolini L, Renda P, Fiore D, Scaglione M, Piccoli G, Giovagnoni A. Acute aortic syndromes: role of multidetector row CT. Eur J Radiol 2008; 65: 350–358.

[20] Estrera AL, Miller CC 3rd, Safi HJ, Goodrick JS, Keyhani A, Porat EE, Achouh PE, Meada R, Azizzadeh A, Dhareshwar J, Allaham A. Outcomes of medical management of acute type B aortic dissection. Circulation 2006; 114(Suppl I): 384–389.

[21] Kodama K, Nishigami K, Sakamoto T, Sawamura T, Hirayama T, Misumi H, Nakao K. Tight heart rate control reduces secondary adverse events in patients with type B acute aortic dissection. Circulation 2008; 118(14 Suppl): S167–S170.

[22] Nienaber CA, Kische S, Rehders TC, Schneider H, Chatterjee T, Bünger CM, Höppner R, Ince H. Rapid pacing for better placing: comparison of techniques for precise deployment of endografts in the thoracic aorta. J Endovasc Ther 2007; 14: 506–512.

[23] Rehders TC, Petzsch M, Ince H, Kische S, Korber T, Koschyk DH, Chatterjee T, Weber F, Nienaber CA. Intentional occlusion of the left subclavian artery during stent-graft implantation in the thoracic aorta: risks and relevance. J Endovasc Ther 2004; 22: 659–666.

[24] Peterson BG, Eskandari MK, Gleason TG, Morasch MD. Utility of left subclavian artery revascularization in association with endoluminal repair of acute and chronic thoracic aortic pathology. J Vasc Surg 2006; 43: 433–439.

[25] Nienaber CA, Kische S, Zeller T, Rehders TC, Schneider H, Lorenzen B, Bünger C, Ince H. Provisional extension to induce complete attachment after stent-graft placement in type B aortic dissection: the PETTICOAT concept. J Endovasc Ther 2006; 13: 738–746.

[26] Schumacher H, von Tengg-Kobligk H, Ostovic M, Henninger V, Ockert S, Böckler D, Allenberg JR. Hybrid arch procedures for endoluminal arch replacement in thoracic aneurysms and type B dissection. J Cardiovasc Surg (Torino) 2006; 47: 509–517.

[27] Saleh HM, Inglese L. Combined surgical and endovascular treatment of aortic arch aneurysms. J Vasc Surg 2006; 44: 460–466.

[28] Czerny M, Gottardi R, Zimpfer D, Schoder M, Grabenwoger M, Lammer J, Wolner E, Grimm M. Transposition of the supraaortic branches for extended endovascular arch repair. Eur J Cardiothorac Surg 2006; 29: 709–713.

[29] Hata M, Shiono M, Inoue T, Sezai A, Niino T, Negishi N, Sezai Y. Optimal treatment of type B acute aortic dissection: long-term medical follow-up results. Ann Thorac Surg 2003; 75: 1781–1784.

[30] Eggebrecht H, Thomson M, Rousseau H, Czerny M, Lönn L, Mehta RH, Erbel R; European Registry on Endovascular Aortic Repair Complications. Retrograde ascending aortic dissection during or after thoracic aortic stent graft placement: insight from the European registry on endovascular aortic repair complications. Circulation 2009; 120(Suppl 11): S276–S281.

[31] Dong ZH, Fu WG, Wang YQ, Guo da Q, Xu X, Ji Y, Chen B, Jiang JH, Yang J, Shi ZY, Zhu T, Shi Y. Retrograde type A aortic dissection after endovascular stent graft placement for treatment of type B dissection. Circulation 2009; 119: 735–741.

Section 5

Abdominal Aortic Aneurysm

Chapter 5

Inflammatory Mediators in Abdominal Aortic Aneurysms

Ismail Cassimjee, Regent Lee and Jyoti Patel

Additional information is available at the end of the chapter

http://dx.doi.org/10.5772/65961

Abstract

Aortic wall dilatation in abdominal aortic aneurysms is characterized by extracellular matrix degradation together with a loss of smooth muscle cells from the aortic media. This occurs in conjunction with a marked inflammatory cell infiltration. The inflammatory cell is characteristic of the second phase of aneurysmal development–progression. It is widely accepted that usually there are three phases involved in the development of abdominal aortic aneurysms: initiation, progression and rupture. In this chapter, we present an overview of the inflammatory mediators in abdominal aortic aneurysms and intraluminal thrombus, highlighting evidence from experimental models and human disease.

Keywords: inflammation, vascular, thrombus, macrophage, T cell

1. Introduction

An abdominal aortic aneurysm (AAA) is an abnormal dilatation of the infrarenal aorta to more than 1.5 times its normal diameter. It poses a risk of rupture which is associated with a significant mortality, and a prophylactic repair is recommended at 5.5 cm in diameter [1–3]. The diameter of an aneurysm is used as a surrogate predictor of rupture risk, and it is at this size that the procedure-related mortality approximates the rupture risk for an overall net benefit in patient survival. There has been much progress in treating aneurysms over the past two decades. The ability to treat aneurysms as minimally invasively, alongside improved perioperative care, has decreased the mortality from elective repair [2—4].

Evidence indicates AAAs as being a disease characterized by an underlying inflammatory cell infiltrate. The inflammatory cell infiltrate consists of differing cell types [macrophages, CD4/CD8 T cells, B cells, natural killer (NK) cells], which interact with each other creating a microenvironment that produces factors, which result in wall degradation as well as further recruitment of other inflammatory cells.

An imbalance in collagen formation and degradation is thought to be responsible for aortic wall rupture [5]. It is a degenerative disease that shares many of the risk factors that predispose a person to atherosclerosis, but it is thought to be a separate pathological process from atherosclerosis (**Table 1**). Atherosclerosis presents typically as an occlusive disease; however, aneurysmal disease is characterized by elastin degeneration and smooth muscle cell apoptosis together with compensatory collagen deposition in the wall of the aneurysm. This may be a result of differing cytokine responses to the underlying inflammatory cell infiltrate [6].

The process of aneurysm formation is complex, and the progression is typically slow. It is multifactorial and requires a combination of anatomical predisposition and common risk factors to trigger its development. The natural history encompasses stages: initiation, formation, growth and rupture [7].

Atherosclerosis	Abdominal aortic aneurysm
Infiltrate through intima	Adventitial inflammation
TH1 predominately early on	TH2 response in the late stages
Diabetes is a significant risk factor	Diabetes may be protective
Stenosing with plaque burden	Dilating with wall rupture
Genetic associations with familial hypercholesterolaemia	Genetic associations with soft tissue degeneration (Col3A1, FBN-1)
Affects both genders equally	Predominantly affects males

TH1: T-helper cell type 1, TH2: T-helper cell type 2.

Table 1. Key differences between atherosclerosis and abdominal aortic aneurysm pathology.

2. Risk factors for AAA development

The development of degenerative AAAs is significantly related to major risk factors such as smoking, advanced age, hypertension and male gender. Having a first-degree relative with an AAA significantly increases the risk of developing an aneurysm. More especially in young patients, there may be an underlying connective tissue disease, like Ehlers-Danlos (Type IV) or Marfan's syndrome. Rarely, inflammatory conditions such as Takayasu's arteritis and Bechet's disease or infective conditions like HIV may present with an aneurysm [4].

3. The aneurysm prone infrarenal aorta

The combination of altered haemodynamics, a different smooth muscle cell derivation and a decrease in the elastic lamella of the infrarenal aorta predisposes it to aneurysm development. The embryological origin of the smooth muscle cells in the aorta of the infrarenal aorta may contribute to aneurysm propensity as they are derived from the splanchnic mesoderm, whereas the arch and thoracic aorta are derived from the neural crest and somite-derived cells, respectively [8]. There is a decrease in the elastin fibre and a decrease in the thickness of the wall of the aorta as it descends from the thorax into the abdominal aorta [9, 10]. In addition, the infrarenal aorta has its maximum number of elastin cells (which produce elastic fibres) at birth [11]. Also, the infrarenal aorta has an increased susceptibility due to reflected pressure waves from the iliac bifurcation leading to a disturbance of the laminar flow and an alteration in the wall shear stress. When compared to the supracoeliac aorta, the infrarenal aorta has, at times, a reversal of flow during diastole, and this can lead to an upregulation of factors that increase the inflammatory infiltrate and proteolytic pathways [12].

4. Mouse models of AAAs

The pathogenesis of AAAs is multifactorial with contributions from a few key risk factors. Aortic tissues received from human subjects reflect a late stage of the disease and may not reflect the early factors involved in initiation. Thus, animal models may provide a better insight into the mechanisms behind aneurysmal degeneration. One of the major advantages of using experimental models of AAA is the ability to knock out or replace endogenous genes, enabling the assessment of the influence of protein expression on the development of disease.

There are several mouse models of chemical-induced AAAs such as elastase infusion into the infrarenal segments of mouse aortas and periaortic administration of calcium chloride between the renal branches and the iliac bifurcation. A more widely used model administers Angiotensin II to induce reproducible AAA. The Angiotensin II-infused mouse model mimics several features of AAAs in humans such as a male gender bias, dilatation of the lumen, degeneration of elastin fibres, inflammatory cell recruitment and thrombus formation [13].

Angiotensin II, a hormone of the renin-angiotensin system, is produced both systemically and locally in the vessel wall [14]. It has diverse actions on signalling pathways that ultimately promote cell growth, proliferation and vascular inflammation [14]. Accordingly, Angiotensin II-induced vascular inflammation can be studied by treating hyperlipidaemic mice with Angiotensin II to investigate long-term chronic inflammatory responses such as plaque formation or short-term acute inflammatory processes such as cellular infiltration. This is thought to occur via activation of the NF-κB cascade, resulting in elevation of cytokines. Furthermore, there is a growing body of evidence that suggests chemokines are involved in the modulation of Angiotensin II-accelerated leucocyte recruitment to the vessel wall [15].

5. Inflammatory cells in AAA

The inflammatory milieu consists of macrophages, monocytes, T cells, NK cells, B cells and other polymorphonuclear cells. They produce various inflammatory factors and mediators, which add to the degradation of collagen, elastin and smooth muscle cells in the aortic wall. The striking histological feature of AAAs is the adventitial and medial inflammatory infiltrate together with medial elastin destruction and fragmentation, and destruction of structural collagens (type 1 and 3) [16, 17]. This excessive elastolysis and collagen destruction are mediated by proteases, most notably the matrix metalloproteases (MMP) family [18]. Several MMPs have been implicated in aneurysm development (MMP-2, 8, 9, 12), with the most evidence for MMP-9 [19]. The other proteases involved are serine proteases (tpa, U-pa, plasmin, neutrophil elastase) and cysteine proteases (Cathepsin D, K, L and S) [16]. The MMPs and the other proteases can be secreted by most of the cells in the aorta (endothelial cells, vascular smooth muscle cells, fibroblasts and macrophages) [16, 20]. MMPs interact closely with tissue inhibitors of MMPs (TIMPS) and these are largely secreted by macrophages, and the process is regulated by cytokines through a feedback loop.

Inflammatory cells occur with a greater frequency in the aneurysmal aorta when compared to the atherosclerotic or non-diseased aorta. The T-cell pattern is different when compared to that of atherosclerotic tissue [21]. The predominant cell types are CD4 T cells, macrophages and B cells [22], and this has led to the assertion that an aortic aneurysm is an inflammatory-mediated condition. It is still not definitively known if the inflammatory cell infiltrate is a cause of, or a reaction to AAAs. It is the microenvironment created by the cellular infiltrate that mediates the production of the proteases that underlie aneurysm progression and probably rupture. One theory suggests that aortic atherosclerosis diverges into aneurysmal formation through a Th2 cytokine response under environmental or genetic stimulation [23].

It has been proposed that an AAA is a specific antigen-driven T-cell disease, where the antigenic specificity remained to be determined [24]. AAA may be an autoimmune disease, and this theory is supported by the following [25]:

1. The presence of mononuclear inflammatory cell infiltrates consisting mainly of T and B cells, macrophages and NK cells [22].
2. Mononuclear cells infiltrating the aneurysm wall show early (CD69), intermediate (CD25, CD38) and late (CD45RO, HLA Class II) activation antigens, suggesting an ongoing inflammation [24].
3. IgG antibody purified from the wall of AAA is immunoreactive with protein derived from normal aortic tissue [26].
4. AAA is associated with particular alleles such as the HLA DRB1 [27].
5. Molecular mimicry may be responsible for T-cell responses in AAA [25].

The pattern of cytokine production by the inflammatory cells influences matrix degradation by regulating their MMP, serine protease and cathepsin production. In murine models of AAA, an IL-4 upregulation and interferon-γ (IFN- γ) blockade together with a predominance of macrophages are the features of early aneurysm formation [23]. The macrophages produce MMP-12, which are stimulated by IL-4 production from T cells, reinforcing the role of IL-4 in early atherosclerosis development [23]. The downstream effects of murine cytokine expression are not always applicable to humans; thus, mechanistic animal studies are difficult to interpret. Also, studies are carried out on tissues *in vitro*, and the complex interaction of the various cytokines is not entirely reproducible [6].

http://dx.doi.org/10.5772/65961

5.1. Macrophages

Macrophages are recruited early into the aneurysmal wall, and macrophage cytokines play an important role in AAA progression. This response is associated with innate immunity as opposed to adaptive immunity. Macrophages exhibit plasticity with regard to their phenotypic cytokine output. They can either be M1 or M2 and can change between the two depending on the prevailing conditions. Typically, M1 macrophages are pro-inflammatory, whereas M2 macrophages are involved in repairing tissue. A balance between M1 and M2 is thus vital in preventing a chronic inflammatory cell infiltrate, which leads to persistent inflammation and aneurysm progression. IL-6, tumour necrosis factor (TNF)-α, IL-1β and interferon (IFN)-γ have been detected peripherally and are associated with aneurysm formation [28].

In murine models of AAA, M1 macrophages are strongly associated with aneurysm formation and elastin degradation; conversely, an M2 phenotype is protective for AAA development [29]. Investigation of human aneurysm tissue has revealed an M1 phenotype, though this tissue represents an end stage of the disease. Most human studies have focused on circulating monocytes and their link to increased elastases and ECM breakdown [30]. ECM breakdown is a recruiter of monocytes, and the use of a monoclonal antibody has been shown to decrease this infiltration and prevent further ECM degradation [31]. Furthermore, the monocytes have demonstrated CD14 and CD16 cell surface marker positivity, and this pattern is associated with M1 macrophage activation [32].

5.2. T cells

As a broad categorization, T cells can be divided up into CD4+ and CD8+ cells. CD4 cells can be further categorized into Th1, Th2, Th17 or regulatory (T_{reg}) cells. This is dependent on drivers of cellular output as well as their cytokine expression. Similar to M1 and M2 macrophages, it would appear that the balance in the different subsets is important for regulation.

Th1 cells are activated by IL-12 and output INF-γ. Aneurysmal tissue displays features of Th1 upregulation with increased INF-γ in the aneurysm tissue and in the circulating blood [28, 33, 34]. Although Th2 cells are found in some specific inflammatory diseases, they are considered to be anti-inflammatory. IL-4 activity is responsible for Th2 differentiation of CD4 T cells, and results are conflicting in murine and human models as to the role of Th2 cells. This discrepancy may be a result of a similar cytokine profile to NK cells (Th0) [35] or from differences in the measurement of the cytokines. Th17 cells produce IL-17, are related to several inflammatory diseases and play a key role in vascular superoxide production [36]. Their role in AAA has not been fully clarified, but they appear to be related to aneurysmal progression.

The frequency of CD4+CD25+FOXP3+ T cells (T_{reg}) is decreased in the peripheral blood of patients with AAA when compared to occlusive atherosclerotic disease or healthy donors [37]. T_{reg} cells are a unique class of T cells that serve as a counter-inflammatory mechanism. In the normal autoregulation of bodily function, there is a balance between T effector cells, which promote inflammation, and T_{reg} cells which counteract this [38]. In inflammatory conditions such as rheumatoid arthritis [39], scleroderma [40], inflammatory bowel disease [41] and transplant organ rejection [42], a dysfunction of Treg cells has been implicated. T_{reg} cells express forkhead box P3 (Foxp3) and are also known as Foxp3+CD4 T cells. They make up approximately 5% of the total CD4+ T cells [43]. The majority of T_{reg} cells express CD25. In the human, T_{reg} cells can be identified by a high expression of CD25 and an absence of IL-7Rα [44].

5.3. Other cell types

Mast cells have been found in the adventitia and media of AAAs and are implicated in AAA formation [45]. They have been found in areas of neovascularization and are able to secrete various cytokines and chemokines. Inhibition of mast cells in experimental mouse models decreases the incidence of aneurysmal formation, furthermore implicating mast cells in the pathogenesis of aneurysms [46]. Neutrophils are early responders to injury and are found in the aneurysm wall as well as the intraluminal thrombus [47]. They interact with many cells including platelets resulting in further inflammatory cell recruitment [48]. In human studies, they have been associated with larger aneurysms, and in animals that are neutrophil deficient, there is a decrease in aneurysm formation [49, 50].

6. Micro-RNAs

Micro-RNAs (miRNA) are a class of non-coding RNA, which are regulators of posttranslational gene expression [51]. They have emerged as potential therapeutic targets due to their ability to control multiple downstream processes. Mir-21 is a regulator of smooth muscle homoeostasis and is upregulated in human as well as animal models of AAA [52]. The mir-29 family encodes multiple ECM targets including elastin and collagen isoforms (type 1 and 3) and fibrillin-1 [53]. Thus, it is important in aneurysm formation. Mir-29b has been found to be downregulated in humans and animal models of AAA as well as in animal models of ageing [54].

7. Intraluminal thrombus (ILT)

The majority of AAAs requiring surgery contain ILT. They are thought to develop secondary to an activated endothelium in combination with disturbances of flow within the aneurysm sac. The volume of ILT is related to growth of the aneurysm, and the thrombus-lined segment of the aorta is structurally different to the non-thrombus-lined area of the aneurysm [55, 56].

There are two major theories on the effect of aneurysmal growth on aortic aneurysm formation. The first relates it to hypoxia of the wall due to the layered thrombus, and the second ascribes it to the inflammatory cell constituents of the thrombus acting in a paracrine manner [57]. The inflammatory cell infiltrate contains macrophages, T cells, granulocytes and NK cells as well as activated platelets [58, 59]. These cells are phenotypically different to the cells found in the wall and the peripheral blood [60]. The exact pathway of interaction between the wall and the ILT has not been fully elucidated, but one theory suggests that microvesicles (ADAM10/ADAM17) shed from the luminal to the abluminal area result in wall breakdown through the formation of elastases in the wall [61].

8. Conclusion

Abdominal aortic aneurysms are regulated by complex and multifactorial processes. At a cellular level, there is a chronic inflammatory cell infiltrate that controls these processes, which lead to growth and rupture. The role of these inflammatory cells has been elegantly demonstrated in experimental models of AAA, and genetic interventions targeting their recruitment and signalling have been known to prevent the development of disease. However, the lack of experimental tools to test the efficacy in human AAA in the preclinical phase and the composition of the thrombus in experimental models has yet to be explored. There has been much work done to understand the inflammatory process, and the hope is that this will lead us to new biomarker discovery and potential therapeutic targets in treating this disease.

Acknowledgements

We would like to acknowledge support from the BHF Centre of Research Excellence, Oxford (RE/13/1/30181).

Author details

Ismail Cassimjee[1], Regent Lee[1] and Jyoti Patel[2, 3]*

*Address all correspondence to: jyoti.patel@well.ox.ac.uk

1 Nuffield Department of Surgery, University of Oxford, UK

2 Division of Cardiovascular Medicine, British Heart Foundation Centre of Research Excellence, University of Oxford, John Radcliffe Hospital, Oxford, UK

3 Wellcome Trust Centre for Human Genetics, University of Oxford, Oxford, UK

References

[1] Powell JT, Greenhalgh RM, Ruckley CV, Fowkes FG. The UK small aneurysm trial. Ann N Y Acad Sci. 1996;800:249–51.

[2] Anderson JL, Halperin JL, Albert NM, Bozkurt B, Brindis RG, Curtis LH, et al. Management of patients with peripheral artery disease (compilation of 2005 and 2011 ACCF/AHA guideline recommendations): a report of the American College of

Cardiology Foundation/American Heart Association Task Force on Practice Guidelines. Circulation. 2013;127(13):1425–43.

[3] Erbel R, Aboyans V, Boileau C, Bossone E, Bartolomeo RD, Eggebrecht H, et al. 2014 ESC Guidelines on the diagnosis and treatment of aortic diseases: document covering acute and chronic aortic diseases of the thoracic and abdominal aorta of the adult. The Task Force for the Diagnosis and Treatment of Aortic Diseases of the European Society of Cardiology (ESC). Eur Heart J. 2014;35(41):2873–926.

[4] Management of Abdominal Aortic Aneurysms Clinical Practice Guidelines of the European Society for Vascular Surgery. 2011;41:S1–S58.

[5] Moll FL, Powell JT, Fraedrich G, Verzini F, Haulon S, Waltham M, et al. Management of abdominal aortic aneurysms clinical practice guidelines of the European society for vascular surgery. Eur J Vasc Endovasc Surg. 2011;41 Suppl 1:S1-s58.

[6] Shimizu K, Libby P, Mitchell RN. Local cytokine environments drive aneurysm formation in allografted aortas. Trends Cardiovasc Med. 2005;15(4):142–8.

[7] Thompson AR, Drenos F, Hafez H, Humphries SE. Candidate gene association studies in abdominal aortic aneurysm disease: a review and meta-analysis. Eur J Vasc Endovasc Surg. 2008;35(1):19–30.

[8] Norman PE, Powell JT. Site specificity of aneurysmal disease. Circulation. 2010;121(4):560–8.

[9] Okuyama K, Yaginuma G, Takahashi T, Sasaki H, Mori S. The development of vasa vasorum of the human aorta in various conditions. A morphometric study. Arch Pathol Lab Med. 1988;112(7):721–5.

[10] Halloran BG, Davis VA, McManus BM, Lynch TG, Baxter BT. Localization of aortic disease is associated with intrinsic differences in aortic structure. J Surg Res. 1995;59(1):17–22.

[11] Kelleher CM, McLean SE, Mecham RP. Vascular extracellular matrix and aortic development. Curr Top Dev Biol. 2004;62:153–88.

[12] Taylor CA, Cheng CP, Espinosa LA, Tang BT, Parker D, Herfkens RJ. In vivo quantification of blood flow and wall shear stress in the human abdominal aorta during lower limb exercise. Ann Biomed Eng. 2002;30(3):402–8.

[13] Trollope A, Moxon JV, Moran CS, Golledge J. Animal models of abdominal aortic aneurysm and their role in furthering management of human disease. Cardiovasc Pathol. 2011;20(2):114–23.

[14] Nguyen Dinh Cat A, Touyz RM. A new look at the renin-angiotensin system–focusing on the vascular system. Peptides. 2011;32(10):2141–50.

[15] Guzik TJ, Hoch NE, Brown KA, McCann LA, Rahman A, Dikalov S, et al. Role of the T cell in the genesis of angiotensin II–induced hypertension and vascular dysfunction. J Exp Med. 2007;204:2449–60.

[16] Liu J, Sukhova GK, Yang JT, Sun J, Ma L, Ren A, et al. Cathepsin L expression and regulation in human abdominal aortic aneurysm, atherosclerosis, and vascular cells. Atherosclerosis. 2006;184(2):302–11.

[17] Galis ZS, Muszynski M, Sukhova GK, Simon-Morrissey E, Unemori EN, Lark MW, et al. Cytokine-stimulated human vascular smooth muscle cells synthesize a complement of enzymes required for extracellular matrix digestion. Circ Res. 1994;75(1):181–9.

[18] Newman KM, Jean-Claude J, Li H, Scholes JV, Ogata Y, Nagase H, et al. Cellular localization of matrix metalloproteinases in the abdominal aortic aneurysm wall. J Vasc Surg. 1994;20(5):814–20.

[19] Lu H, Rateri DL, Bruemmer D, Cassis LA, Daugherty A. Novel mechanisms of abdominal aortic aneurysms. Curr Atheroscler Rep. 2012;14(5):402–12.

[20] Knox JB, Sukhova GK, Whittemore AD, Libby P. Evidence for altered balance between matrix metalloproteinases and their inhibitors in human aortic diseases. Circulation. 1997;95(1):205–12.

[21] Schönbeck U, Sukhova GK, Gerdes N, Libby P. TH2 predominant immune responses prevail in human abdominal aortic aneurysm. Am J Pathol. 2002;161(2):499–506.

[22] Koch AE, Haines GK, Rizzo RJ, Radosevich JA, Pope RM, Robinson PG, et al. Human abdominal aortic aneurysms. Immunophenotypic analysis suggesting an immune-mediated response. Am J Pathol. 1990;137(5):1199–213.

[23] Shimizu K, Mitchell RN, Libby P. Inflammation and cellular immune responses in abdominal aortic aneurysms. Arterioscler Thromb Vasc Biol. 2006;26(5):987–94.

[24] Platsoucas CD, Lu S, Nwaneshiudu I, Solomides C, Agelan A, Ntaoula N, et al. Abdominal aortic aneurysm is a specific antigen-driven T cell disease. Ann N Y Acad Sci. 2006;1085:224–35.

[25] Lu S, White JV, Lin WL, Zhang X, Solomides C, Evans K, et al. Aneurysmal lesions of patients with abdominal aortic aneurysm contain clonally expanded T cells. J Immunol. 2014;192(10):4897–912.

[26] Xia S, Ozsvath K, Hirose H, Tilson MD. Partial amino acid sequence of a novel 40-kDa human aortic protein, with vitronectin-like, fibrinogen-like, and calcium binding domains: aortic aneurysm-associated protein-40 (AAAP-40) [human MAGP-3, proposed]. Biochem Biophys Res Commun. 1996;219(1):36–9.

[27] Rasmussen TE, Hallett JW, Jr., Metzger RL, Richardson DM, Harmsen WS, Goronzy JJ, et al. Genetic risk factors in inflammatory abdominal aortic aneurysms: polymorphic residue 70 in the HLA-DR B1 gene as a key genetic element. J Vasc Surg. 1997;25(2):356–64.

[28] Juvonen J, Surcel HM, Satta J, Teppo AM, Bloigu A, Syrjala H, et al. Elevated circulating levels of inflammatory cytokines in patients with abdominal aortic aneurysm. Arterioscler Thromb Vasc Biol. 1997;17(11):2843–7.

[29] Dale MA, Xiong W, Carson JS, Suh MK, Karpisek AD, Meisinger TM, et al. Elastin-derived peptides promote abdominal aortic aneurysm formation by modulating M1/M2 macrophage polarization. J Immunol. 2016;196(11):4536–43.

[30] Samadzadeh KM, Chun KC, Nguyen AT, Baker PM, Bains S, Lee ES. Monocyte activity is linked with abdominal aortic aneurysm diameter. J Surg Res. 2014;190(1):328–34.

[31] Hance KA, Tataria M, Ziporin SJ, Lee JK, Thompson RW. Monocyte chemotactic activity in human abdominal aortic aneurysms: role of elastin degradation peptides and the 67-kD cell surface elastin receptor. J Vasc Surg. 2002;35(2):254–61.

[32] Ghigliotti G, Barisione C, Garibaldi S, Brunelli C, Palmieri D, Spinella G, et al. CD16(+) monocyte subsets are increased in large abdominal aortic aneurysms and are differentially related with circulating and cell-associated biochemical and inflammatory biomarkers. Dis Markers. 2013;34(2):131–42.

[33] Galle C, Schandene L, Stordeur P, Peignois Y, Ferreira J, Wautrecht JC, et al. Predominance of type 1 CD4+ T cells in human abdominal aortic aneurysm. Clin Exp Immunol. 2005;142(3):519–27.

[34] Liao M, Xu J, Clair AJ, Ehrman B, Graham LM, Eagleton MJ. Local and systemic alterations in signal transducers and activators of transcription (STAT) associated with human abdominal aortic aneurysms. J Surg Res. 2012;176(1):321–8.

[35] Chan WL, Pejnovic N, Liew TV, Hamilton H. Predominance of Th2 response in human abdominal aortic aneurysm: mistaken identity for IL-4-producing NK and NKT cellsγ Cell Immunol. 2005;233(2):109–14.

[36] Madhur MS, Funt SA, Li L, Vinh A, Chen W, Lob HE, et al. Role of interleukin 17 in inflammation, atherosclerosis, and vascular function in apolipoprotein e-deficient mice. Arterioscler Thromb Vasc Biol. 2011;31(7):1565–72.

[37] Yin M, Zhang J, Wang Y, Wang S, Bockler D, Duan Z, et al. Deficient CD4+CD25+ T regulatory cell function in patients with abdominal aortic aneurysms. Arterioscler Thromb Vasc Biol. 2010;30(9):1825–31.

[38] Dale MA, Ruhlman MK, Baxter BT. Inflammatory cell phenotypes in AAAs: their role and potential as targets for therapy. Arterioscler Thromb Vasc Biol. 2015;35(8):1746–55.

[39] Ehrenstein MR, Evans JG, Singh A, Moore S, Warnes G, Isenberg DA, et al. Compromised function of regulatory T cells in rheumatoid arthritis and reversal by anti-TNFalpha therapy. J Exp Med. 2004;200(3):277–85.

[40] Venigalla RK, Tretter T, Krienke S, Max R, Eckstein V, Blank N, et al. Reduced CD4+,CD25γ T cell sensitivity to the suppressive function of CD4+, CD25high, CD127γ/low regulatory T cells in patients with active systemic lupus erythematosus. Arthritis Rheum. 2008;58(7):2120–30.

[41] Uhlig HH, Coombes J, Mottet C, Izcue A, Thompson C, Fanger A, et al. Characterization of Foxp3+CD4+CD25+ and IL-10-secreting CD4+CD25+ T cells during cure of colitis. J Immunol. 2006;177(9):5852–60.

[42] Sumpter TL, Wilkes DS. Role of autoimmunity in organ allograft rejection: a focus on immunity to type V collagen in the pathogenesis of lung transplant rejection. Am J Physiol Lung Cell Mol Physiol. 2004;286(6):L1129–39.

[43] Zhou Y, Wu W, Lindholt JS, Sukhova GK, Libby P, Yu X, et al. Regulatory T cells in human and angiotensin II-induced mouse abdominal aortic aneurysms. Cardiovasc Res. 2015;107(1):98–107.

[44] Zhu J, Paul WE. CD4 T cells: fates, functions, and faults. Blood. 2008;112(5):1557–69.

[45] Mayranpaa MI, Trosien JA, Fontaine V, Folkesson M, Kazi M, Eriksson P, et al. Mast cells associate with neovessels in the media and adventitia of abdominal aortic aneurysms. J Vasc Surg. 2009;50(2):388–95; discussion 95–6.

[46] Sun J, Sukhova GK, Yang M, Wolters PJ, MacFarlane LA, Libby P, et al. Mast cells modulate the pathogenesis of elastase-induced abdominal aortic aneurysms in mice. J Clin Invest. 2007;117(11):3359–68.

[47] Houard X, Ollivier V, Louedec L, Michel JB, Back M. Differential inflammatory activity across human abdominal aortic aneurysms reveals neutrophil-derived leukotriene B4 as a major chemotactic factor released from the intraluminal thrombus. Faseb J. 2009;23(5):1376–83.

[48] Houard X, Touat Z, Ollivier V, Louedec L, Philippe M, Sebbag U, et al. Mediators of neutrophil recruitment in human abdominal aortic aneurysms. Cardiovasc Res. 2009;82(3):532–41.

[49] Eliason JL, Hannawa KK, Ailawadi G, Sinha I, Ford JW, Deogracias MP, et al. Neutrophil depletion inhibits experimental abdominal aortic aneurysm formation. Circulation. 2005;112(2):232–40.

[50] Ramos-Mozo P, Madrigal-Matute J, Martinez-Pinna R, Blanco-Colio LM, Lopez JA, Camafeita E, et al. Proteomic analysis of polymorphonuclear neutrophils identifies catalase as a novel biomarker of abdominal aortic aneurysm: potential implication of oxidative stress in abdominal aortic aneurysm progression. Arterioscler Thromb Vasc Biol. 2011;31(12):3011–9.

[51] Maegdefessel L, Dalman RL, Tsao PS. Pathogenesis of abdominal aortic aneurysms: microRNAs, proteases, genetic associations. Annu Rev Med. 2014;65:49–62.

[52] Maegdefessel L, Azuma J, Toh R, Deng A, Merk DR, Raiesdana A, et al. MicroRNA-21 blocks abdominal aortic aneurysm development and nicotine-augmented expansion. Sci Transl Med. 2012;4(122):122ra22.

[53] van Rooij E, Sutherland LB, Liu N, Williams AH, McAnally J, Gerard RD, et al. A signature pattern of stress-responsive microRNAs that can evoke cardiac hypertrophy and heart failure. Proc Natl Acad Sci USA. 2006;103(48):18255–60.

[54] Boon RA, Seeger T, Heydt S, Fischer A, Hergenreider E, Horrevoets AJ, et al. MicroRNA-29 in aortic dilation: implications for aneurysm formation. Circ Res. 2011;109(10):1115–9.

[55] Stenbaek J, Kalin B, Swedenborg J. Growth of thrombus may be a better predictor of rupture than diameter in patients with abdominal aortic aneurysms. Eur J Vasc Endovasc Surg. 2000;20(5):466–9.

[56] Kazi M, Johan T, Religa P, Roy J, Eriksson P. Influence of intraluminal thrombus on structural and cellular composition of abdominal aortic aneurysm wall. J Vasc Surg. 2003;38(6):1283–92.

[57] Vorp DA, Lee PC, Wang DH, Makaroun MS, Nemoto EM, Ogawa S, et al. Association of intraluminal thrombus in abdominal aortic aneurysm with local hypoxia and wall weakening. J Vasc Surg. 2001;34(2):291–9.

[58] Adolph R, Vorp DA, Steed DL, Webster MW, Kameneva MV, Watkins SC. Cellular content and permeability of intraluminal thrombus in abdominal aortic aneurysm. J Vasc Surg. 1997;25(5):916–26.

[59] Sagan A, Mrowiecki W, Mikolajczyk TP, Urbanski K, Siedlinski M, Nosalski R, et al. Local inflammation is associated with aortic thrombus formation in abdominal aortic aneurysms. Relationship to clinical risk factors. Thromb Haemost. 2012;108(5):812–23.

[60] Rao J, Brown BN, Weinbaum JS, Ofstun EL, Makaroun MS, Humphrey JD, et al. Distinct macrophage phenotype and collagen organization within the intraluminal thrombus of abdominal aortic aneurysm. J Vasc Surg. 2015;62(3):585–93.

[61] Folkesson M, Li C, Frebelius S, Swedenborg J, Wagsater D, Williams KJ, et al. Proteolytically active ADAM10 and ADAM17 carried on membrane microvesicles in human abdominal aortic aneurysms. Thromb Haemost. 2015;114(6): 1165–1174.

Chapter 6

Sexual Dimorphism of Abdominal Aortic Aneurysms

Yasir Alsiraj, Sean E. Thatcher and Lisa A. Cassis

Additional information is available at the end of the chapter

http://dx.doi.org/10.5772/64611

Abstract

Sex is the largest nonmodifiable risk factor for the development of abdominal aortic aneurysms (AAAs) in humans and experimental models. Data from several studies consistently demonstrate a higher AAA prevalence in males than in females, contributing to divergent recommendations for AAA screening in men and women. Despite a higher AAA prevalence in males, females have more rapid rates of aneurysm dilation, and aneurysms rupture at smaller sizes. Unfortunately, no therapies have been effective to retard aneurysm dilation in either sex. Results from experimental AAA models indicate a protective role for estrogen in AAA development and progression, while male testosterone has been demonstrated to markedly promote angiotensin II (AngII)-induced AAAs. Potential mechanisms implicated in sex hormone regulation of AAAs include regulation of inflammation, matrix metalloproteinases, aromatase activity, oxidative stress, stem cells, and transforming growth factor-beta. In addition to sex hormones, sex chromosomes have been implicated in diseases of the aorta. Turner's syndrome (monosomy X) patients have a high incidence of thoracic aortic rupture. Recent studies indicate a novel approach to define the relative role of sex hormones versus sex chromosomes in experimental AAAs. Further studies are warranted to determine interactions between sex hormones and sex chromosomes in AAA development and progression.

Keywords: sex chromosomes, sex hormones, gender, AAA

1. Introduction

As defined by the Society of Vascular Surgery, abdominal aortic aneurysms (AAAs) are a permanent dilation of the infrarenal aorta (ratio of ≥1.5-fold increase in normal abdominal aortic diameter) [1], leading to infrarenal aortic diameters >3 cm that can expand to more than 5.5 cm [2]. AAAs are typically asymptomatic, which is of concern due to the high mortality rate from aneurysm rupture. The prevalence of asymptomatic AAAs in geriatric men and women ranged from 4 to 14.2% and from 0.35 to 6.2%, respectively [3–5]. Between the ages of 50 and 84 years, it has been estimated that AAA prevalence could be as high as 1.1 million people in the United States [6]. AAAs are responsible for 1.3% of all deaths in men between the ages of 65 and 85 years [7]. According to the Society of Vascular Surgery, in the United States, there are 200,000 people diagnosed with an AAA each year, and it is the 10th leading cause of mortality in men more than 55 years of age [8]. Impending rupture of AAAs is associated with sudden, severe, and constant groin, abdominal, and lower back pain. Because the aorta is the main supplier of blood throughout the body, AAA rupture can result in fatal bleeding with 85% chance of death. Depending on AAA expansion rate and size, treatment might vary from frequent monitoring (typically by ultrasound) to open or endovascular aneurysm repair. As AAA size increases (diameter > 5.5 cm), the probability of rupture also increases. While age, smoking, male sex, and family history are positively associated with AAA development, female sex, smoking cessation, and a healthy diet are negatively associated with AAA formation [6].

2. Sex differences in AAA prevalence in human and experimental models

Sex is considered a strong nonmodifiable risk factor for AAA formation. The incidence of AAAs has been reported to range from 4- to 5-fold higher in men compared to women [9, 10], with studies indicating that men are at a 10-fold higher risk to develop AAA compared to age-matched women [10]. Results from the Tromsø Study demonstrate that male sex contributes a 2.66 relative risk for AAA formation [11]. Epidemiological studies have shown an increased AAA incidence and rupture in men originating from western countries [12, 13]. In a community-based older population screening study, it was found that the AAA prevalence was 1.3% in women in comparison to 7.6% in men [14]. Correspondingly, the male:female ratio in a surgical series was ≈5:1. Hospitalization for ruptured or intact AAA was 5 times more prevalent among men than women [9]. After controlling for time of surgery and age, men were around 1.8 times as likely to have an intact AAA treated surgically and 1.4 times to have a ruptured AAA in comparison to women. Current screening recommendations are to screen annually by ultrasound for men between the ages of 65 and 75 years with either a family history of AAA or who smoke. Conversely, studies have also shown that female sex decreases the AAA risk [10]. These results indicate that across a broad range of large-scale clinical trials, AAAs are much more prevalent in men as compared to women. In addition to male sex, the most predominant risk factors for AAAs are age, smoking, and family history.

Even though women have far lower AAA prevalence compared to men, women have worse prognosis than men, as AAAs in women progress faster and rupture at smaller sizes [15, 16]. Using the Vascular Study Group of New England database, Lo et al. have shown that women are older when diagnosed with an AAA, have smaller aortic diameters, and stay in the hospital longer than men diagnosed with an intact AAA [17]. Furthermore, women more frequently experience complications (e.g., leg and bowel ischemia) and have a higher mortality after 30 days than men after open AAA repair [17]. Also, according to the National Service hospitals in England, all cause and aortic-related mortalities were higher in women at all-time points (30 days, 1 year, and 5 years) in both open and EVAR surgeries [18]. Additional studies have shown that the survival rate in women after surgical repair is lower than that of men; however, mechanisms for these effects are largely undefined [19, 20]. Differences in AAA rupture and progression between men and women could relate to vascular anatomy. For example, Lo and Schermerhorn noted that if the ratio of infrarenal to suprarenal diameter is ≥1.2 or a definition of ≥1.5 times the normal aortic diameter, then AAA prevalence in women could be as high as 6.2–9.8% [21]. This would indicate that using the same vascular anatomic criteria for men and women could lead to underdiagnosis of small AAAs in women [21]. While there is general consensus that men should be screened at 65 years of age or older, only the Society for Vascular Surgery recommends screening women (65 or older) who have smoked or have a family history of AAA [21]. In fact, some studies have indicated that women who smoke are more likely than nonsmoking men to develop AAAs [22]. An additional area of concern relates to recommendations for endovascular aneurysm repair as women having this procedure with a small AAA have poor outcomes (and also for open AAA repair) [17, 18]. Another issue related to the use of endovascular aneurysm repair in women is poor access to smaller vessels. These access-related complications lead to arterial injury of vessels which may result in additional surgeries and/or problems with stent engraftment.

In addition to anatomical differences, aortic wall stress differs between men and women. A recent study analyzed biomechanical and microstructural properties of nonaneurysmal human male and female aortas and concluded that male aortas are stiffer than female aortas [23]. Male aortas had higher failure load and tension than female aortas [23], which was suggested as a mechanism explaining rupture of AAAs in women at smaller sizes. Additionally, a small study (15 women and 15 men) examined peak wall stress (PWS) and peak wall rupture risk (PWRR) of AAA between men and women. Using computed tomography (CT) scans, results did not support differences in PWS between men and women; however, there was a trend for higher PWRR in females [24]. Future studies should utilize CT imaging to determine if criteria such as PWRR are informative for AAA diagnosis and in defining AAA growth.

An interesting study examined 140 Swedish women with an AAA compared to the same number of women with peripheral arterial disease (non-AAA) [25]. Results demonstrated smoking as a risk factor for AAA while diabetes was protective, but an interesting aspect of this study was the segregation of women who had an AAA ≥5 cm versus <5 cm that showed differences in onset of menopause. Women who had large AAAs were approximately 2 years younger at age for menopause than those women who had smaller AAAs [25]. These data suggest that ovarian hormones may play a role in protection from large AAA development.

In addition to humans, experimental AAA models also exhibit sexual dimorphism, and have been used to define mechanisms of AAA formation and progression. Depending on the experimental model under study, AAAs recapitulate several facets of the human disease including medial degeneration, thrombus formation, and inflammation. The majority of experimental AAA models are evoked by genetic and/or chemical interventions, including increased degradation of collagen and elastin, defects in extracellular matrix maturation, aberrant cholesterol homeostasis, increased aldosterone, and salt levels, as well as enhanced generation of or exposure to angiotensin peptides [26–30]. Similar to humans, male mice infused with angiotensin II (AngII) exhibit a 4-fold higher prevalence of AAAs compared to female mice [31].

Typically, AAA incidence in male, hypercholesterolemic mice is 80% with females having a much lower incidence (20%) [31]. Our laboratory demonstrated previously that sex hormones are primary contributors to higher AAA susceptibility in male compared to female apoliproprotein E deficient (*Apoe*$^{-/-}$) mice, as ovariectomy had no effect on AAA formation while orchiectomy decreased AAA incidence to the level of females [31, 32]. We also demonstrated that testosterone promotes AAA incidence in male and female mice associated with increased expression of angiotensin receptor 1a (AT1aR) expression specifically in abdominal aortas [32]. Similarly, in the elastase perfusion AAA model, male rats had larger and more frequent AAAs than females [33].

3. Influences of sex hormones on AAA development and progression

Limited studies have examined effects of sex hormone replacement therapy (HRT) in relation to AAA development, while experimental studies have focused primarily on therapeutics of sex hormones. Use of HRT for greater than 5 years in women decreased the odds ratio of developing an AAA [34]. However, other studies have shown no beneficial effect of HRT on AAA outcomes [35, 36]. Castration of male mice decreased AAA development and progression in both elastase and AngII-induced models [31–33, 37, 38]. In contrast, castration of female mice did not influence AAA development in either of these models [31, 37]. However, another study demonstrated ovariectomy of Wistar rats promoted elastase-induced AAAs [39].

In addition to effects of endogenous sex hormones, exogenous administration of estrogen inhibited AAA development and/or progression in AngII-infused male mice, while exogenous dihydrotestosterone administration also promoted AngII-induced AAAs in females [32, 37, 39–42]. Mechanisms of estrogen to protect against AAA formation and/or progression are multifactorial. Inflammation is frequently associated with AAAs [43], and recent studies demonstrated that peripheral blood monocytes contained sex and disease-specific inflammasome signatures that could be potential biomarkers to determine which patients may have AAAs [44].

In experimental AAAs, results demonstrated that estrogen replacement in ovariectomized female low density lipoprotein receptor deficient mice (*Ldlr*$^{-/-}$) decreased neutrophil AAA content [40]. Also, exogenous estrogen administration to AngII-infused male *Apoe*$^{-/-}$ mice decreased nuclear factor-kappa B (NF-kappa B) activity and immune cell adhesion markers in the aorta [42]. Dietary phytoestrogens have also been demonstrated to decrease inflammation and AAA formation in elastase-induced male mice [45]. Plasmin activator inhibitor-1 (PAI-1) expression was increased in aortas from elastase-perfused female mice compared to males, while PAI whole body deficiency enhanced AAA development in both sexes [46].

An additional mechanism evoked in sex hormone effects on AAA development and/or progression is regulation of matrix metalloproteinase (MMP) activity. Results demonstrate that aortas from elastase-perfused female rats and mice have lower MMP activity than males [33, 47]. Likewise, ovariectomy of female Wistar rats increased aortic MMP-2 and -9 activity [39]. Conversely, administration of estrogen to male rats decreased aortic MMP-2 or MMP-9 activity compared to vehicle controls [33, 48]. An ability of estrogen to regulate MMP activity differs according to the experimental model understudy, as estrogen incubations in rat aortic smooth muscle cells (SMCs) did not alter MMP-2 activity, while estrogen stimulated MMP activity in aortic explants [48].

Oxidative stress has also been implicated as a mechanism for sex hormone regulation of AAAs. Superoxide dismutase (SOD) is an enzyme that converts superoxide radical to either oxygen or hydrogen peroxide. Deletion of SOD abolished sex differences in myogenic tone of mesenteric arteries from male compared to female mice [49]. Additional studies demonstrated that SMCs harvested from male and female rat aortas respond differently to ultraviolet B (UVB)-induced radiation [50]. Male SMCs were shown to produce more superoxide anion and SOD levels were lower in SMCs from male than female mice [50]. UVB-induced radiation resulted in apoptosis of SMCs that was also greater in male compared to female mice [50]. Interestingly, nitric oxide regulates SOD levels, but results using a carotid injury model demonstrated that males increase SOD levels in response to nitric oxide whereas females do not [51]. A recent study demonstrated that UVB-induced radiation resulted in upregulation of survival proteins in the nucleus of SMCs from female rats, but increased proapoptotic proteins and reduced mitochondrial membrane potential in SMCs from males [52].

Differences in estrogen formation and signaling such as aromatase activity and levels of estrogen receptors (ERs) could also contribute to sex differences in AAAs. Deletion of aromatase abolished the protective effects of female gender on elastase-induced AAAs [53]. Aortas from female mice had higher expression levels of ER α compared to male mice by day 3 of elastase perfusion [47]. Increased ERα expression was also detected in female human AAA patients compared to males [47]. Tamoxifen, a selective estrogen receptor modulator, decreased AAA development in male rats associated with decreased aortic neutrophil content, MMP-9 activity, and oxidative stress [54].

Sex differences have also been found in transforming growth factor-beta (TGF-β) and other members of the bone morphogenetic protein family (BMPs) related to AAA development [40, 55]. Elastase-perfused aortas from female rats had decreased TGF-β expression compared to males [55]. Moreover, exposure of murine SMCs to exogenous estrogen increased TGF-β expression and enhanced wound healing [40]. Deletion of the androgen receptor (AR) in either macrophages or SMCs lowered TGF-β1 expression levels and suppressed AAA development in male mice [56]. In contrast, antibody-based depletion of TGF-β increased AAA ruptures in male mice [57, 58]. Mechanisms for these discrepancies are unclear, but may relate to sex hormones, sex chromosomes, or an interplay thereof [59].

Recent studies indicate that bone marrow-derived mesenchymal stem cells (MSCs) exhibit sex-dependent effects that influence AAA development [60]. When female MSCs were injected into male mice, elastase-induced AAAs were attenuated [60]. Furthermore, when conditioned media from MSCs was injected (i.v.) to male mice AAA formation was attenuated [60]. Moreover, the 5-alpha-reductase inhibitor, finasteride, decreased proinflammatory cytokine expression in male MSCs [60]. In humans, endothelial progenitor cells from AAA patients are impaired [61]. Taken together, these studies suggest that stem cells may have therapeutic potential for AAAs depending on patient sex.

In addition to protective effects in females, results indicate that male sex hormones may have detrimental effects on AAA formation and/or progression. For example, high levels of luteinizing hormone were positively associated with AAA outcomes [62]. Interestingly, lower testosterone levels have been linked to coronary artery disease and peripheral arterial disease in older men, but show little association when grouped with younger men [63–65].

Previous studies in our laboratory demonstrated that testosterone is a primary mediator of higher AAA prevalence in adult AngII-infused male mice, as orchiectomy decreased AAA incidence to the level of adult females [32]. Additional studies demonstrated a greater abundance of AT1aR mRNA in abdominal compared to thoracic aortas of male, but not female *Apoe*$^{-/-}$ mice [32]. Moreover, castration of male mice decreased AT1aR mRNA abundance in abdominal aortas, which was restored when castrated male mice were administered dihydrotestosterone [32]. Administration of dihydrotestosterone to female mice also increased abdominal aortic AT1aR mRNA abundance, and promoted AngII-induced AAAs. To explore mechanisms contributing to regional differences in AT1aR abundance along the aortic length, we initiated studies examining developmental influences of testosterone. The rationale for these studies was based on diversity of SMC origin along the aortic length [66], coupled with expression of AR in abdominal aortic SMCs derived from mesenchymal stem cells [67]. Using a novel model whereby neonatal female mice were exposed to a single dose of testosterone (e.g., to mimic testosterone surges after birth in males), we demonstrated a robust increase in adult AAA susceptibility in females that was associated with increased abdominal aortic AT1aR expression [31, 32]. Since increased abdominal aortic AT1aR mRNA abundance and high AAA susceptibility persisted in adult females exposed transiently to testosterone during development despite a low-level of circulating testosterone, these results indicate that the simple presence of testosterone does not define sex differences in AAA susceptibility. Finally, in addition to influencing AAA formation, recent studies from our laboratory demonstrated that castration of male *Apoe*$^{-/-}$ mice after an AAA was established halted progressive increases in abdominal aortic lumen diameter but had no effect on maximal AAA diameters [38]. Castration of male mice was associated with increased aortic wall rigidity through increases in collagen and smooth muscle α-actin [38].

As an alternative approach to administering exogenous sex hormone, genetic deficiency of AR decreased elastase-induced AAA formation in male mice associated with decreasing aortic mRNA abundance of proinflammatory cytokines IL-1α, IL-6, and IL-17 [68]. In different studies, whole body AR deficiency in male *Apoe*$^{-/-}$ mice was demonstrated to suppress IL-1α expression in aortic tissue, while AngII infusion stimulated aortic IL-1α expression in wild type male controls [56]. Deletion of the AR specifically from macrophages or SMCs decreased AngII-induced AAAs in male *Apoe*$^{-/-}$ mice that could be partially restored by administering recombinant IL-1α [56]. Male mice have increased abdominal aortic IL-1β mRNA and protein levels when perfused with elastase [69], and increased levels of c-Jun-N-terminal kinase (JNK), proMMP-9, proMMP-2, and active MMP-2 [70]. While it is unclear if these sex differences relate to testosterone, results consistently indicate differences in aortic inflammatory pathways that may contribute to sexual dimorphism of AAAs.

Several sex hormone-mediated effects that may relate to AAA development have been demonstrated in SMCs. For example, testosterone stimulated oxidative stress of SMCs harvested from

http://dx.doi.org/10.5772/64611

male mice [41]. Moreover, SMCs harvested from male mice exhibited increased MMP-2 and 9 activity and AKT phosphorylation [71], increased levels of phosphorylated extracellular signal-regulated kinase (p-Erk), and elevated proMMP-2 levels when exposed to elastase [72]. Male SMCs exhibit increased levels of MMP-2 compared to female rats when stimulated with IL-1β [48]. Additionally, MMP-9 mRNA abundance was 10-fold higher in male compared to female SMCs.

4. Potential influence of sex chromosomes on AAA development

Sex chromosomes can also contribute to sexually dimorphic responses of the cardiovascular system [73]. However, as described above, sexual dimorphism of AAAs has primarily been attributed to direct or indirect effects of sex hormones, even though sex hormones do not fully explain all sexual dimorphism. Studies have shown that there are large sex differences of gene expression in somatic tissues of mice [74]. Sex hormones are known to be important in differentiation of the reproductive system and also impact sex differences in gene expression in somatic tissues. However, differences in pregonadal embryo size between males and females are also influenced by sex chromosome complement [75, 76]. Moreover, before gonadal differentiation, a large number of genes are expressed differentially in preimplantation embryos [77]. These results indicate that sex chromosome genes in addition to sex hormone regulation influence development.

Beyond their effects on sex determination and reproduction, there is little known about the role of genes residing on sex chromosomes in disease development, especially in the vasculature. The sex chromosomes are designated as X and Y. In mammals, there are 23 pairs of chromosomes, one pair of sex chromosomes that are either XX or XY, and 22 pairs of autosomes. The Y chromosome is responsible for sex determination, because it has the Sex determining Region of the Y (Sry) gene that resides in the male-specific region of the Y chromosome (MSY). The MSY represents 95% of Y chromosome content and does not recombine with the X chromosome during meiosis. This region of the Y chromosome is responsible for testis formation; however, if the Sry gene is absent, the fetus will be female even in the presence of the Y chromosome. The Sry gene has been demonstrated to regulate the expression of several components of the renin-angiotensin system. It has been shown that Sry increases the promoter activity for angiotensinogen, renin, and angiotensin-converting enzyme 1 (ACE1) and decreases angiotensin-converting enzyme 2 (ACE2) promoter activity in Chinese Hamster Ovary (CHO) cells [78]. It is unclear if these effects are related to sex differences in AAAs and/or other cardiovascular diseases associated with an activated renin-angiotensin system.

The sex chromosomes do not recombine normally like autosomes; they usually recombine at their tips which are called pseudoautosomal regions (homologous regions of nucleotides sequences that recombine with each other during meiosis). The most important characteristic feature of sex chromosomes is that the Y chromosome is missing a large number of genes compared to the X chromosome. As a result, male and female cells have a different dosage of X and Y genes that could influence cell function differently in gonadal and nongonadal tissues.

In addition to sex hormones, genes present on the sex chromosomes are thought to be a primary mechanism for differences between males and females. While the Y chromosome is small and has few genes, the X chromosome is large and contains 1098 genes [79]. X-linked genes, including components of the renin-angiotensin system such as ACE2 and angiotensin type 2 receptors (AT2R), are present in males and females, but two X chromosomes in females can cause gene-dosage differences for X-linked genes between males and females. The possible difference in expression of genes on the X chromosome is typically compensated for by X chromosome inactivation, in which one of the two X chromosomes becomes silenced transcriptionally. However, some genes escape X-inactivation, or are differentially expressed depending on which X chromosome is inactivated (maternal or paternal) and can lead to gene-dosage effects between XX and XY cells.

Genes on sex chromosomes have been linked to inherited forms of cardiovascular diseases [80, 81], but it is still unclear what role sex chromosomes and their interaction with sex hormones have on the development of these diseases. Recently, an experimental study demonstrated that the numbers of X chromosomes influences protection from cardiac ischemia, because mice with two X chromosomes were more vulnerable to myocardial infarction when compared to mice with one X and one Y chromosome [82]. Klinefelter syndrome (47 XXY), the most common abnormality of sex chromosomes in males due to the presence of an extra X chromosome, is associated with increased cardiovascular risk and mortality [83, 84]. Turner syndrome (45X) in females, or monosomy X (XO), is a common chromosomal disorder that is due to partial or complete loss of one of the X chromosomes. Females with Turner syndrome exhibit a 100-fold increased risk of aortic dissection [85]. These results suggest that sex chromosome complement can influence the vasculature, but mechanisms for these effects are unknown.

AAAs are also an aortic disease that can be genetically inherited [86–89]. First degree relatives of AAA patients are at 11.6-fold higher risk of developing aneurysmal degeneration compared to non-AAA families [86]. Moreover, in a multinational study that investigated a large number of families, each family that contained at least two individuals with a diagnosed AAA were predominately male (77% of patients) and the most common relationship was being a male sibling [90]. Since the Y chromosome is passed only from father to son, this suggests a potential role for the Y chromosome in male AAA susceptibility. However, despite the strong predisposition for AAA formation in males compared to females, the contribution of sex chromosome effects to AAA inheritance and sexual dimorphism of this vascular disease has not been explored.

Since XX chromosomes are most commonly presented in nature with ovaries (females) while XY chromosomes exist in males with testes, previously it has not been possible to examine the role of sex chromosome complement independent of gonadal hormone effects in experimental animal models. However, there are now experimental models, such as the four core genotype model in mice, which can be used to understand the relative influence of sex chromosomes in the absence or presence of gonadal hormones. The four core genotype model is produced from male mice with a natural mutation of Sry, where this gene was reinserted on autosomes. Breeding of male mice with autosomal Sry to females produces four genotypes, XX and XY females (with ovaries) and XY and XX males (with testes) [91]. Recent studies using this model identified that blood pressure responses to infusion of AngII were influenced by both sex hormones and sex chromosomes, as blood pressure responses to AngII were greater in gonadectomized XX than XY females [92]. Furthermore, vasodilation of iliac arteries was greater in XX than XY females and this effect appeared to be AT2R-dependent [93].

Since sex chromosome complement also influences the blood pressure response to AngII, it is highly likely that sex chromosome effects on gene expression influence other AngII-mediated responses, such as AAAs. Moreover, uncovering the basic knowledge of the interplay between sex hormones and sex chromosomes on aortic vascular biology and disease may lead to discovery of novel drug targets that have efficacy in a sex-specific manner.

5. Summary

It is clear that AAAs are sexually dimorphic in prevalence and prognosis. The majority of studies defining mechanisms for sexual dimorphism of AAAs have focused on potential roles for sex hormones (see **Table 1** for summary), with estrogen generally thought to be protective while testosterone exerts detrimental effects that promote AAA formation and progression. However, given a strong inheritance for AAAs, coupled with an association of sex chromosome abnormalities with aortic vascular disease, additional studies defining potential roles for sex chromosome genes in AAA development are warranted.

Gender	Study [Ref.]	Model	Intervention	Effect on AAA
Males	Martin-McNulty et al. [42]	AngII-induced AAA in mice	17 Beta-estradiol administration	Decrease
Males	Henriques et al. [31]	AngII-induced AAA in mice	Orchidectomy	Decrease
Males	Grigoryants et al. [54]	Elastase perfusion in rats	Tamoxifen (selective estrogen receptor modulators) administration	Decrease
Males	Laser et al. [47]	Elastase perfusion in mice	Low ERα expression	High AAA
Males	Zhang et al. [38]	AngII-induced AAA in mice	Orchidectomy	Decrease the progression of established AngII-induced AAAs
Males	Cho et al. [37]	Elastase perfusion in rats	Estrogen administration or orchiectomy	Decrease AAA diameter
Males	Huang et al. [56]	AngII-induced AAA in mice	ASC-J19 (androgen receptor degradation enhancer)	Decrease
Males	Huang et al. [56]	AngII-induced AAA in mice	Androgen receptor knockout in macrophage or smoth muscle cells	Decrease
Males	Huang et al. [56]	AngII-induced AAA in mice	Androgen receptor knockout in endothelial cells	No effect
Males	Davis et al. [68]	Elastase perfusion in mice	Flutamide (androgen receptor blocker)	Decrease
Males	Davis et al. [68]	Elastase perfusion in mice	Ketoconazole (androgen receptor blocker)	Decrease

Gender	Study [Ref.]	Model	Intervention	Effect on AAA
Males	Davis et al. [68]	Elastase perfusion in mice	Deletion of androgen receptor	Decrease
Females	Cho et al. [37]	Elastase perfusion in rats	Testosterone administration or oophorectomy	No effect
Females	Zhang et al. [41]	AngII-induced AAA in mice	Neonatal testosterone administration	Increase
Females	Laser et al. [47]	Elastase perfusion in mice	High ERα expression	Low AAA
Females	Thatcher et al. [40]	AngII-induced AAA in mice	17 Beta-estradiol administration	Decrease the progression of established AngII-induced AAA in ovariectomized females
Females and Males	Laser et al. [47]	Human	ERα protein level	ERα protein levels 80% higher in female human AAA patients than those in male counterparts
Females and Males	Johnston et al. [53]	Elastase perfusion in mice	Aromatase knockout	Increase in females and no effect in males

Table 1. Influence of sex hormone manipulation on experimental AAAs.

Acknowledgements

We acknowledge funding from the National Institutes of Health (HL107326).

Author details

Yasir Alsiraj, Sean E. Thatcher and Lisa A. Cassis*

*Address all correspondence to: lcassis@uky.edu

Department of Pharmacology and Nutritional Sciences, University of Kentucky, Lexington, KY, USA

References

[1] Johnston KW, Rutherford RB, Tilson MD, Shah DM, Hollier L, Stanley JC. Suggested standards for reporting on arterial aneurysms. Subcommittee on reporting standards for arterial aneurysms, ad hoc committee on reporting standards, society for vascular surgery and North American chapter, international society for cardiovascular surgery. J Vasc Surg. 1991;13(3):452–8.

[2] Jamrozik K, Spencer CA, Lawrence-Brown MM, Norman PE. Does the Mediterranean paradox extend to abdominal aortic aneurysm? Int J Epidemiol. 2001;30(5):1071–5.

[3] Lawrence-Brown MM, Norman PE, Jamrozik K, Semmens JB, Donnelly NJ, Spencer C, et al. Initial results of ultrasound screening for aneurysm of the abdominal aorta in Western Australia: relevance for endoluminal treatment of aneurysm disease. Cardiovasc Surg. 2001;9(3):234–40.

[4] Cornuz J, Sidoti Pinto C, Tevaearai H, Egger M. Risk factors for asymptomatic abdominal aortic aneurysm: systematic review and meta-analysis of population-based screening studies. Eur J Public Health. 2004;14(4):343–9.

[5] Palombo D, Lucertini G, Pane B, Mazzei R, Spinella G, Brasesco PC. District-based abdominal aortic aneurysm screening in population aged 65 years and older. J Cardiovasc Surg (Torino). 2010;51(6):777–82.

[6] Kent KC, Zwolak RM, Egorova NN, Riles TS, Manganaro A, Moskowitz AJ, et al. Analysis of risk factors for abdominal aortic aneurysm in a cohort of more than 3 million individuals. J Vasc Surg. 2010;52(3):539–48.

[7] Sakalihasan N, Limet R, Defawe OD. Abdominal aortic aneurysm. Lancet. 2005;365(9470):1577–89.

[8] Singh M. Abdominal aortic aneurysm [webpage]. Society for Vascular Surgery; 2016 [Available from: {http://vascular.org/patient-resources/vascular-conditions/abdominal-aortic-aneurysm}.

[9] Katz DJ, Stanley JC, Zelenock GB. Gender differences in abdominal aortic aneurysm prevalence, treatment, and outcome. J Vasc Surg. 1997;25(3):561–8.

[10] Lederle FA, Johnson GR, Wilson SE, Aneurysm D, Management veterans affairs cooperative S. Abdominal aortic aneurysm in women. J Vasc Surg. 2001;34(1):122–6.

[11] Forsdahl SH, Singh K, Solberg S, Jacobsen BK. Risk factors for abdominal aortic aneurysms: a 7-year prospective study: the Tromso Study, 1994–2001. Circulation. 2009;119(16):2202–8.

[12] Acosta S, Ogren M, Bengtsson H, Bergqvist D, Lindblad B, Zdanowski Z. Increasing incidence of ruptured abdominal aortic aneurysm: a population-based study. J Vasc Surg. 2006;44(2):237–43.

[13] Best VA, Price JF, Fowkes FG. Persistent increase in the incidence of abdominal aortic aneurysm in Scotland, 1981–2000. Br J Surg. 2003;90(12):1510–5.

[14] Scott RA, Bridgewater SG, Ashton HA. Randomized clinical trial of screening for abdominal aortic aneurysm in women. Br J Surg. 2002;89(3):283–5.

[15] Brown LC, Powell JT. Risk factors for aneurysm rupture in patients kept under ultrasound surveillance. UK Small Aneurysm Trial Participants. Ann Surg. 1999;230(3):289–96; discussion 96-7.

[16] Brown PM, Zelt DT, Sobolev B. The risk of rupture in untreated aneurysms: the impact of size, gender, and expansion rate. J Vasc Surg. 2003;37(2):280–4.

[17] Lo RC, Bensley RP, Hamdan AD, Wyers M, Adams JE, Schermerhorn ML, et al. Gender differences in abdominal aortic aneurysm presentation, repair, and mortality in the Vascular Study Group of New England. J Vasc Surg. 2013;57(5):1261–8, 8 e1–5.

[18] Desai M, Choke E, Sayers RD, Nath M, Bown MJ. Sex-related trends in mortality after elective abdominal aortic aneurysm surgery between 2002 and 2013 at National Health Service hospitals in England: less benefit for women compared with men. Eur Heart J. 2016:1–9.

[19] Noel AA, Gloviczki P, Cherry KJ, Jr., Bower TC, Panneton JM, Mozes GI, et al. Ruptured abdominal aortic aneurysms: the excessive mortality rate of conventional repair. J Vasc Surg. 2001;34(1):41–6.

[20] Norman PE, Powell JT. Abdominal aortic aneurysm: the prognosis in women is worse than in men. Circulation. 2007;115(22):2865–9.

[21] Lo RC, Schermerhorn ML. Abdominal aortic aneurysms in women. J Vasc Surg. 2016;63(3):839–44.

[22] Stackelberg O, Bjorck M, Larsson SC, Orsini N, Wolk A. Sex differences in the association between smoking and abdominal aortic aneurysm. Br J Surg. 2014;101(10):1230–7.

[23] Ninomiya OH, Tavares Monteiro JA, Higuchi Mde L, Puech-Leao P, de Luccia N, Raghavan ML, et al. Biomechanical properties and microstructural analysis of the human nonaneurysmal aorta as a function of age, gender and location: An autopsy study. J Vasc Res. 2015;52(4):257–64.

[24] Larsson E, Labruto F, Gasser TC, Swedenborg J, Hultgren R. Analysis of aortic wall stress and rupture risk in patients with abdominal aortic aneurysm with a gender perspective. J Vasc Surg. 2011;54(2):295–9.

[25] Villard C, Swedenborg J, Eriksson P, Hultgren R. Reproductive history in women with abdominal aortic aneurysms. J Vasc Surg. 2011;54(2):341–5, 5 e1–2.

[26] Daugherty A, Manning MW, Cassis LA. Angiotensin II promotes atherosclerotic lesions and aneurysms in apolipoprotein E-deficient mice. J Clin Invest. 2000;105(11):1605–12.

[27] Halpern VJ, Nackman GB, Gandhi RH, Irizarry E, Scholes JV, Ramey WG, et al. The elastase infusion model of experimental aortic aneurysms: synchrony of induction of endogenous proteinases with matrix destruction and inflammatory cell response. J Vasc Surg. 1994;20(1):51–60.

[28] Carrell TW, Smith A, Burnand KG. Experimental techniques and models in the study of the development and treatment of abdominal aortic aneurysm. Br J Surg. 1999;86(3):305–12.

[29] Takayanagi T, Crawford KJ, Kobayashi T, Obama T, Tsuji T, Elliott KJ, et al. Caveolin 1 is critical for abdominal aortic aneurysm formation induced by angiotensin II and inhibition of lysyl oxidase. Clin Sci (Lond). 2014;126(11):785–94.

[30] Liu S, Xie Z, Daugherty A, Cassis LA, Pearson KJ, Gong MC, et al. Mineralocorticoid receptor agonists induce mouse aortic aneurysm formation and rupture in the presence of high salt. Arterioscler Thromb Vasc Biol. 2013;33(7):1568–79.

[31] Henriques TA, Huang J, D'Souza SS, Daugherty A, Cassis LA. Orchidectomy, but not ovariectomy, regulates angiotensin II-induced vascular diseases in apolipoprotein E-deficient mice. Endocrinology. 2004;145(8):3866–72.

[32] Henriques T, Zhang X, Yiannikouris FB, Daugherty A, Cassis LA. Androgen increases AT1a receptor expression in abdominal aortas to promote angiotensin II-induced AAAs in apolipoprotein E-deficient mice. Arterioscler Thromb Vasc Biol. 2008;28(7):1251–6.

[33] Ailawadi G, Eliason JL, Roelofs KJ, Sinha I, Hannawa KK, Kaldjian EP, et al. Gender differences in experimental aortic aneurysm formation. Arterioscler Thromb Vasc Biol. 2004;24(11):2116–22.

[34] Lederle FA, Larson JC, Margolis KL, Allison MA, Freiberg MS, Cochrane BB, et al. Abdominal aortic aneurysm events in the women's health initiative: cohort study. BMJ. 2008;337:a1724.

[35] Hsia J, Criqui MH, Rodabough RJ, Langer RD, Resnick HE, Phillips LS, et al. Estrogen plus progestin and the risk of peripheral arterial disease: the Women's Health Initiative. Circulation. 2004;109(5):620–6.

[36] Hsia J, Criqui MH, Herrington DM, Manson JE, Wu L, Heckbert SR, et al. Conjugated equine estrogens and peripheral arterial disease risk: the women's health initiative. Am Heart J. 2006;152(1):170–6.

[37] Cho BS, Woodrum DT, Roelofs KJ, Stanley JC, Henke PK, Upchurch GR, Jr. Differential regulation of aortic growth in male and female rodents is associated with AAA development. J Surg Res. 2009;155(2):330–8.

[38] Zhang X, Thatcher S, Wu C, Daugherty A, Cassis LA. Castration of male mice prevents the progression of established angiotensin II-induced abdominal aortic aneurysms. J Vasc Surg. 2015;61(3):767–76.

[39] Wu XF, Zhang J, Paskauskas S, Xin SJ, Duan ZQ. The role of estrogen in the formation of experimental abdominal aortic aneurysm. Am J Surg. 2009;197(1):49–54.

[40] Thatcher SE, Zhang X, Woody S, Wang Y, Alsiraj Y, Charnigo R, et al. Exogenous 17-beta estradiol administration blunts progression of established angiotensin II-induced abdominal aortic aneurysms in female ovariectomized mice. Biol Sex Differ. 2015;6:12.

[41] Zhang X, Thatcher SE, Rateri DL, Bruemmer D, Charnigo R, Daugherty A, et al. Transient exposure of neonatal female mice to testosterone abrogates the sexual dimorphism of abdominal aortic aneurysms. Circ Res. 2012;110(11):e73–85.

[42] Martin-McNulty B, Tham DM, da Cunha V, Ho JJ, Wilson DW, Rutledge JC, et al. 17 Beta-estradiol attenuates development of angiotensin II-induced aortic abdominal aneurysm in apolipoprotein E-deficient mice. Arterioscler Thromb Vasc Biol. 2003;23(9):1627–32.

[43] Hellmann DB, Grand DJ, Freischlag JA. Inflammatory abdominal aortic aneurysm. JAMA. 2007;297(4):395–400.

[44] Wu X, Cakmak S, Wortmann M, Hakimi M, Zhang J, Bockler D, et al. Sex- and disease-specific inflammasome signatures in circulating blood leukocytes of patients with abdominal aortic aneurysm. Mol Med. 2016;22(22):508–18.

[45] Lu G, Su G, Zhao Y, Johnston WF, Sherman NE, Rissman EF, et al. Dietary phytoestrogens inhibit experimental aneurysm formation in male mice. J Surg Res. 2014;188(1):326–38.

[46] DiMusto PD, Lu G, Ghosh A, Roelofs KJ, Su G, Zhao Y, et al. Increased PAI-1 in females compared with males is protective for abdominal aortic aneurysm formation in a rodent model. Am J Physiol Heart Circ Physiol. 2012;302(7):H1378–86.

[47] Laser A, Ghosh A, Roelofs K, Sadiq O, McEvoy B, DiMusto P, et al. Increased estrogen receptor alpha in experimental aortic aneurysms in females compared with males. J Surg Res. 2014;186(1):467–74.

[48] Woodrum DT, Ford JW, Cho BS, Hannawa KK, Stanley JC, Henke PK, et al. Differential effect of 17-beta-estradiol on smooth muscle cell and aortic explant MMP2. J Surg Res. 2009;155(1):48–53.

[49] Veerareddy S, Cooke CL, Baker PN, Davidge ST. Gender differences in myogenic tone in superoxide dismutase knockout mouse: animal model of oxidative stress. Am J Physiol Heart Circ Physiol. 2004;287(1):H40–5.

[50] Malorni W, Straface E, Matarrese P, Ascione B, Coinu R, Canu S, et al. Redox state and gender differences in vascular smooth muscle cells. FEBS Lett. 2008;582(5):635–42.

[51] Morales RC, Bahnson ES, Havelka GE, Cantu-Medellin N, Kelley EE, Kibbe MR. Sex-based differential regulation of oxidative stress in the vasculature by nitric oxide. Redox Biol. 2015;4:226–33.

[52] Straface E, Vona R, Campesi I, Franconi F. Mitochondria can orchestrate sex differences in cell fate of vascular smooth muscle cells from rats. Biol Sex Differ. 2015;6:34.

[53] Johnston WF, Salmon M, Su G, Lu G, Ailawadi G, Upchurch GR, Jr. Aromatase is required for female abdominal aortic aneurysm protection. J Vasc Surg. 2015;61(6):1565–74 e1–4.

[54] Grigoryants V, Hannawa KK, Pearce CG, Sinha I, Roelofs KJ, Ailawadi G, et al. Tamoxifen up-regulates catalase production, inhibits vessel wall neutrophil infiltration, and attenuates development of experimental abdominal aortic aneurysms. J Vasc Surg. 2005;41(1):108–14.

[55] Sinha I, Cho BS, Roelofs KJ, Stanley JC, Henke PK, Upchurch GR, Jr. Female gender attenuates cytokine and chemokine expression and leukocyte recruitment in experimental rodent abdominal aortic aneurysms. Ann N Y Acad Sci. 2006;1085:367–79.

[56] Huang CK, Luo J, Lai KP, Wang R, Pang H, Chang E, et al. Androgen receptor promotes abdominal aortic aneurysm development via modulating inflammatory interleukin-1alpha and transforming growth factor-beta1 expression. Hypertension. 2015;66(4):881–91.

[57] Wang Y, Ait-Oufella H, Herbin O, Bonnin P, Ramkhelawon B, Taleb S, et al. TGF-beta activity protects against inflammatory aortic aneurysm progression and complications in angiotensin II-infused mice. J Clin Invest. 2010;120(2):422–32.

[58] Chen X, Rateri DL, Howatt DA, Balakrishnan A, Moorleghen JJ, Cassis LA, et al. TGF-beta Neutralization Enhances AngII-Induced Aortic Rupture and Aneurysm in Both Thoracic and Abdominal Regions. PLoS One. 2016;11(4):e0153811.

[59] Wang Y, Krishna S, Walker PJ, Norman P, Golledge J. Transforming growth factor-beta and abdominal aortic aneurysms. Cardiovasc Pathol. 2013;22(2):126–32.

[60] Davis JP, Salmon M, Pope NH, Lu G, Su G, Sharma AK, et al. Attenuation of aortic aneurysms with stem cells from different genders. J Surg Res. 2015;199(1):249–58.

[61] Sung SH, Wu TC, Chen JS, Chen YH, Huang PH, Lin SJ, et al. Reduced number and impaired function of circulating endothelial progenitor cells in patients with abdominal aortic aneurysm. Int J Cardiol. 2013;168(2):1070–7.

[62] Yeap BB, Hyde Z, Norman PE, Chubb SA, Golledge J. Associations of total testosterone, sex hormone-binding globulin, calculated free testosterone, and luteinizing hormone with prevalence of abdominal aortic aneurysm in older men. J Clin Endocrinol Metab. 2010;95(3):1123–30.

[63] Chan YX, Knuiman MW, Hung J, Divitini ML, Handelsman DJ, Beilby JP, et al. Testosterone, dihydrotestosterone and estradiol are differentially associated with carotid intima-media thickness and the presence of carotid plaque in men with and without coronary artery disease. Endocr J. 2015;62(9):777–86.

[64] Tivesten A, Mellstrom D, Jutberger H, Fagerberg B, Lernfelt B, Orwoll E, et al. Low serum testosterone and high serum estradiol associate with lower extremity peripheral arterial disease in elderly men. The MrOS Study in Sweden. J Am Coll Cardiol. 2007;50(11):1070–6.

[65] Chan YX, Knuiman MW, Hung J, Divitini ML, Beilby JP, Handelsman DJ, et al. Neutral associations of testosterone, dihydrotestosterone and estradiol with fatal and non-fatal cardiovascular events, and mortality in men aged 17-97 years. Clin Endocrinol (Oxf). 2016;85(4): 575–82.

[66] Majesky MW. Developmental basis of vascular smooth muscle diversity. Arterioscler Thromb Vasc Biol. 2007;27(6):1248–58.

[67] Cunha GR, Shannon JM, Neubauer BL, Sawyer LM, Fujii H, Taguchi O, et al. Mesenchymal-epithelial interactions in sex differentiation. Hum Genet. 1981;58(1):68–77.

[68] Davis JP, Salmon M, Pope NH, Lu G, Su G, Meher A, et al. Pharmacologic blockade and genetic deletion of androgen receptor attenuates aortic aneurysm formation. J Vasc Surg. 2016;63(6):1602–12 e2.

[69] Johnston WF, Salmon M, Su G, Lu G, Stone ML, Zhao Y, et al. Genetic and pharmacologic disruption of interleukin-1beta signaling inhibits experimental aortic aneurysm formation. Arterioscler Thromb Vasc Biol. 2013;33(2):294–304.

[70] DiMusto PD, Lu G, Ghosh A, Roelofs KJ, Sadiq O, McEvoy B, et al. Increased JNK in males compared with females in a rodent model of abdominal aortic aneurysm. J Surg Res. 2012;176(2):687–95.

[71] Ghosh A, Lu G, Su G, McEvoy B, Sadiq O, DiMusto PD, et al. Phosphorylation of AKT and abdominal aortic aneurysm formation. Am J Pathol. 2014;184(1):148–58.

[72] Ehrlichman LK, Ford JW, Roelofs KJ, Tedeschi-Filho W, Futchko JS, Ramacciotti E, et al. Gender-dependent differential phosphorylation in the ERK signaling pathway is associated with increased MMP2 activity in rat aortic smooth muscle cells. J Surg Res. 2010;160(1):18–24.

[73] Arnold AP. Mouse models for evaluating sex chromosome effects that cause sex differences in non-gonadal tissues. J Neuroendocrinol. 2009;21(4):377–86.

[74] Yang X, Schadt EE, Wang S, Wang H, Arnold AP, Ingram-Drake L, et al. Tissue-specific expression and regulation of sexually dimorphic genes in mice. Genome Res. 2006;16(8):995–1004.

[75] Thornhill AR, Burgoyne PS. A paternally imprinted X chromosome retards the development of the early mouse embryo. Development. 1993;118(1):171–4.

[76] Burgoyne PS, Thornhill AR, Boudrean SK, Darling SM, Bishop CE, Evans EP. The genetic basis of XX-XY differences present before gonadal sex differentiation in the mouse. Philos Trans R Soc Lond B Biol Sci. 1995;350(1333):253–60 discussion 60–1.

[77] Bermejo-Alvarez P, Rizos D, Rath D, Lonergan P, Gutierrez-Adan A. Sex determines the expression level of one third of the actively expressed genes in bovine blastocysts. Proc Natl Acad Sci U S A. 2010;107(8):3394–9.

[78] Milsted A, Underwood AC, Dunmire J, DelPuerto HL, Martins AS, Ely DL, et al. Regulation of multiple renin-angiotensin system genes by Sry. J Hypertens. 2010;28(1):59–64.

[79] Ross MT, Grafham DV, Coffey AJ, Scherer S, McLay K, Muzny D, et al. The DNA sequence of the human X chromosome. Nature. 2005;434(7031):325–37.

[80] Bloomer LD, Nelson CP, Eales J, Denniff M, Christofidou P, Debiec R, et al. Male-specific region of the Y chromosome and cardiovascular risk: phylogenetic analysis and gene expression studies. Arterioscler Thromb Vasc Biol. 2013;33(7):1722–7.

[81] Charchar FJ, Tomaszewski M, Strahorn P, Champagne B, Dominiczak AF. Y is there a risk to being male? Trends Endocrinol Metab. 2003;14(4):163–8.

[82] Li J, Chen X, McClusky R, Ruiz-Sundstrom M, Itoh Y, Umar S, et al. The number of X chromosomes influences protection from cardiac ischaemia/reperfusion injury in mice: one X is better than two. Cardiovasc Res. 2014;102(3):375–84.

[83] Bojesen A, Gravholt CH. Morbidity and mortality in Klinefelter syndrome (47,XXY). Acta Paediatr. 2011;100(6):807–13.

[84] Bojesen A, Juul S, Birkebaek N, Gravholt CH. Increased mortality in Klinefelter syndrome. J Clin Endocrinol Metab. 2004;89(8):3830–4.

[85] Wong SC, Cheung M, Zacharin M. Aortic dilatation and dissection in Turner syndrome: what we know, what we are unclear about and what we should do in clinical practice? Int J Adolesc Med Health. 2014;26(4):469–88.

[86] Johansen K, Koepsell T. Familial tendency for abdominal aortic aneurysms. JAMA. 1986;256(14):1934–6.

[87] Blanchard JF, Armenian HK, Friesen PP. Risk factors for abdominal aortic aneurysm: results of a case-control study. Am J Epidemiol. 2000;151(6):575–83.

[88] Clifton MA. Familial abdominal aortic aneurysms. Br J Surg. 1977;64(11):765–6.

[89] Rossaak JI, Hill TM, Jones GT, Phillips LV, Harris EL, van Rij AM. Familial abdominal aortic aneurysms in the Otago region of New Zealand. Cardiovasc Surg. 2001;9(3):241–8.

[90] Kuivaniemi H, Shibamura H, Arthur C, Berguer R, Cole CW, Juvonen T, et al. Familial abdominal aortic aneurysms: collection of 233 multiplex families. J Vasc Surg. 2003;37(2):340–5.

[91] Itoh Y, Mackie R, Kampf K, Domadia S, Brown JD, O'Neill R, et al. Four core genotypes mouse model: localization of the Sry transgene and bioassay for testicular hormone levels. BMC Res Notes. 2015;8:69.

[92] Ji H, Zheng W, Wu X, Liu J, Ecelbarger CM, Watkins R, et al. Sex chromosome effects unmasked in angiotensin II-induced hypertension. Hypertension. 2010;55(5):1275–82.

[93] Pessoa BS, Slump DE, Ibrahimi K, Grefhorst A, van Veghel R, Garrelds IM, et al. Angiotensin II type 2 receptor- and acetylcholine-mediated relaxation: essential contribution of female sex hormones and chromosomes. Hypertension. 2015;66(2):396–402.

Chapter 7

Endograft Sizing for Abdominal Aortic Aneurysms

Alex Sher and Rami O. Tadros

Additional information is available at the end of the chapter

http://dx.doi.org/10.5772/66369

Abstract

While a tight seal and fixation of aortic stent-grafts to the vessel wall are vital for positive outcomes in treating abdominal aortic aneurysms (AAAs), optimal aortic stent-graft sizing for endovascular aneurysm repair (EVAR) remains debatable. We performed a holistic review of the data surrounding the sizing of endografts using instructions for use (IFU) guidelines, as well as experimental, computational, and clinical studies. Most clinical studies that have investigated the role of sizing and outcomes are limited by the strict selection criteria, or the inability to account for the multitude of confounders associated with sizing. Currently, oversizing of endografts between 10 and 20% remains safe and favored, but sizing outside the IFU guidelines frequently occurs. Oversizing up to 25% appears to be associated with decreased rates of proximal endoleak and aneurysm sac enlargement, while excessive oversizing (>30%) has been linked to graft infolding, collapse, and aortic dilatation. It is unclear, however, whether there is an association between oversizing associated with neck dilatation and graft migration. During sizing, surgeons should take an individual approach and consider several factors including device type, calcification and/or thrombus of apposition site, hemodynamics, and aortoiliac morphology.

Keywords: endovascular aneurysm repair, sizing, endograft, instructions for use, abdominal aortic aneurysm

1. Introduction

Aortic aneurysms, a ballooning of a weakened portion of the aorta, are most frequently seen in the abdominal aorta. When indicated, an abdominal aortic aneurysm (AAA) can be treated with open surgical or endovascular repair. With a higher perioperative morbidity and mortality of open surgery [1–6], endovascular aneurysm repair (EVAR) of the abdominal aorta has grown in popularity as a safe, effective, and minimally invasive alternative for certain patients. The goal of EVAR is to achieve adequate fixation and to seal the stent graft to the vessel wall, thus redirecting blood flow away from the pathologic section of the aorta n/a. Failure to do so can result in several noteworthy complications, including device migration or kinking, dilatation, and most commonly perigraft endoleak. In fact, some have reported endoleak complications in up to 20–25% of patients following the EVAR [7, 8]. Ultimately, these complications can lead to occlusion of adjacent branches, aneurysm sac growth, or even rupture.

Exploration of the use of nonporous endoprosthesis for the treatment of AAA dates back to 1976, when Parodi et al. [9] began to transform Dacron prosthetics into intraluminal devices. Several others went on to test the intraluminal grafts in animals with an array of sizing protocols [10–13]. However, it is difficult to interpret sizing practices from these early studies since most involved balloon-expandable stents and not the self-expandable stents that are frequently used today. Since the approval of self-expandable aortic stent-grafts in humans with AAAs over a decade ago, sizing has become a crucial component of the successful EVAR. Early feasibility studies recommended sizing the device larger than the vessel (i.e., oversizing) without strong scientific backing. After years of use, evidence for oversizing has been validated [14, 15]. Oversizing helps in securing the device in place and achieving adequate fixation and seal by increasing the frictional force between the vessel and device. Additionally, oversizing addresses the unevenness of each vessel and allows the vessel to take the circular shape of the device [16]. Ultimately, the device must generate a large enough radial force to resist displacement from the vessel wall, but not so large that the endograft starts to fold or cause adverse vessel remodeling.

Although most surgeons agree about the importance of sizing, several factors make it a difficult task. For one, angulated vessels may introduce variability in the degree of oversizing delivered around the vessel wall. Others include the presence of thrombus or calcification at the attachment sites, length and shape of apposition sites, graft features, and stability of vessels. Further complicating, sizing is the reality that the pulsatility of vessels and hemodynamics of each patient is variable. Nevertheless, the instructions for use (IFU) guidelines of most devices recommend sizing the endovascular graft 10–20% larger than the vessel diameter. However, these sizing recommendations lack comparable safety and effectiveness studies for aortic grafts sized outside that range. Moreover, graft oversizing in patients frequently varies from the manufacturer's IFU, with reported oversizing ranging from less than 5% to greater than 40% [17]. With this variability, and because the complication rate post EVAR remains significant, the optimal degree of oversizing continues to be a topic of interest for many surgeons.

2. Aim of the chapter

The aim of this chapter is to provide physicians with a useful resource when sizing stent-grafts for EVAR of the abdominal aorta. This chapter provides the instructions for use guidelines published by each graft manufacturer and objectively reviews the relationship between the endograft sizing and outcomes using experimental, computational, and clinical studies.

http://dx.doi.org/10.5772/66369

3. Early development and sizing

The difficulty of sizing prosthesis can be seen as early as the implantation of sutureless intraluminal grafts during open surgery. With the goal of better fixation, Matsumae et al. [18] proposed the addition of elastic rings and saw no dislodgment or migration in nine canines with a ratio of 0.92–0.70 (31.4%) of ring to aorta diameter. In 1983, Nitinol wires were inserted in animals using a transluminal approach with only the stent dimensions reported [19, 20]. Since wires were not a feasible solution to exclude the aneurysm sac, several attempts were made testing intraluminal grafts in animals [9–13]. Balko et al. [10] used 10 mm intraluminal polyurethane prosthesis with a compressible Nitinol wire frame in a 9 mm self-made aneurysm in sheep. Laborde et al. [13] used 10 mm modified tubular Dacron grafts affixed to balloon-expandable stents and applied it to 10 mm mongrel vessels and found inconsistent results; yet, they recommended expanding the stent to a diameter 10–15% larger than the aorta. In 1991, Parodi et al. [9] achieved a "watertight seal" in humans using a balloon-expandable stent, but unfortunately, the sizing of each patient was not reported. Soon after, several studies investigated the anatomy of patients with AAA in order to identify the range of endograft sizes necessary for treatment [21, 22]. Thus, the importance of accurately sizing endografts was clear early on. Manufacturers of these early grafts recommended that stent-grafts should be oversized a few millimeters. It is not clear, however, what scientific observations were used to make these recommendations. Even in 1999, an experimental study reported that they supported the "theoretical" advantage of oversizing prosthesis [15]. Nevertheless, these early feasibility studies highlight how oversizing has been an important part of EVAR since the early development.

4. Endograft devices and instructions for use

Since the first device implanted in patients in 1991, several modifications have been made with efforts to address access, fixation, and sealing. Devices can be classified as either balloon- or self-expandable. The most commonly used devices today are self-expandable and they have the advantage of providing more anatomically correct support. The manufacturers of approved endografts suggest measuring either from intima to intima (inner wall) or adventitia to adventitia (outer wall). Thus, when deciding how much to oversize, the apposition site diameter measurements should be device-specific. The following consists of a brief timeline of the currently available self-expandable devices.

In 1999, the Food and Drug Administration (FDA) first approved the use of two self-expandable endografts, the AneuRx (Medtronic Vascular, Santa Rosa, CA, USA) and Ancure (Guidant Corporation, Indianapolis, IN, USA). Yet, by 2001, Guidant suspended the production and announced the recall of all Ancure devices. In 2002 and 2003, respectively, the Excluder (W.L. Gore & Associates, Flagstaff, AZ, USA) and Zenith (Cook Inc., Bloomington, IN, USA) devices gained approval. More recently, the Powerlink (Endologix, Irvine, CA, USA), Talent (Medtronic, Inc., Minneapolis, MN, USA), and Endurant (Medtronic, Inc., Minneapolis, MN, USA) devices were all approved. The characteristics of each device currently available along with their recommended sizing protocols are given below (**Table 1**). The associated exclusion criteria, study designs, and outcomes from their clinical trials are also summarized (**Table 2**). Of note, the anatomical requirements for inclusion in these studies are often strict and do not represent the scope of patients currently being treated with EVAR. Thus, the anatomical characteristics of each study should be considered when evaluating the degree of oversizing used. Finally, by proving safety and effectiveness, many of these studies helped in guiding the recommendations for the endograft sizing today. What they did not show, however, was the effect of different levels of sizing on outcomes. In general, the instructions for use recommendations suggest using an individual approach and oversizing stent-grafts 10–20% in the abdominal aorta with a wider accepted range of up to 25% in the iliac arteries.

Device	Design	Active fixation	Suprarenal or infrarenal	Available sizes	Sizing recommendation
AneuRx (Medtronic, Inc.)	Modular, bifurcated, Nitinol stent, polyster fabric	No	Infrarenal	Main body: 20–28 mm, iliac limb: 12–24 mm	Approximately 2 mm larger than the aortic diameter and 1 mm larger iliac diameter (10–20% oversizing)—see IFU
Excluder (W.L. Gore & Associates, Inc.)	Modular, bifurcated, Nitinol stent, ePTFE fabric	Yes (anchors)	Infrarenal	Main body: 23–31 mm, iliac limb: 10–20 mm	At least 2 mm larger than the aortic inner diameter (10–21% oversizing) and 1 mm larger than the iliac inner diameter (7–25% oversizing)—see IFU
Zenith (Cook Medical, Inc.)	Modular, bifurcated, stainless steel Z-stents, polyster Dacron fabric	Yes (barbs)	Suprarenal	Main body: 22–36 mm, iliac limb: 8–24 mm	Varying based on outer diameter aortic: (14–24%) iliac: (0–20%)—see IFU
Powerlink (Endologix)	Modular, bifurcated unibody, cobalt chromium stent, ePTFE	No	Infrarenal	Main body: 25–28 mm, iliac limb: 16 mm, extenstion limb: 16–25 mm	Varying based on diameter—see IFU
Talent (Medtronic, Inc.)	Modular, bifurcated, nitinol stent, polyster fabric	No	Suprarenal	Main body: 22–36 mm, iliac limb: 8–24 mm	Varying based on diameter aortic: (14–24%) iliac: (0–20%)—see IFU
Endurant (Medtronic, Inc.)	Modular, bifurcated or aorta-uniiliac, Nitinol M-shaped stent, high filament polyster fabric	Yes (pins)	Suprarenal	Main body: 23–36 mm, iliac limb: 10–28 mm	Aorta: 10–20% larger than vessel inner diameter iliac: 10–25% larger than vessel inner diameter—see IFU

ePTFE, expanded polytetrafluoroethylene.

Table 1. Characteristics of commercially available self-expandable aortic stent-grafts.

http://dx.doi.org/10.5772/66369

Device	FDA approval	Clinical study sizing	Study design	N	Follow-up	Patients excluded	Anatomical characteristics	Outcomes
AneuRx	1999	Not specified (recommended 10–20% overisizing)	Nonrandomized, prospective, multicenter clinical study	416	6 months, 1 year	• Aneurysmal neck or proximal neck length <10 mm • Infrarenal neck diameter <18 mm or >26 mm • Neck angluation >60° • Iliac diameter >16 mm • Iliac landing zone length <15 mm • Vessel morphology not suitable for endovascular repair	• Median neck diameter 20–29 mm • Median aneurysm diameter 50–59 mm	**Migration** Predischarge—baseline 6 months—1.7% 1 year—1.6% **Endoleak (any)** Predischarge—43.8% 6 months—24% 1 year—17.4%
Excluder/low permeability excluder*	2002/2004	Not specified (recommended 10–21% overisizing aorta and 7–25% iliacs)	Nonrandomized prospective, multicenter clinical studies	563/139*	1 month, 6 months, 1 year, 2 years, 3 years, 4 years, 5 years	• Infrarenal proximal neck lengh <15 mm • Infrarenal aneurysmal aortic neck or diameter > 29 mm • Proximal neck angulation >60° • Presence of significant thrombus at implantation sites • Iliac and femoral arteries not suitable for EVAR • Vessel morphology not suitable for endovascular repair	• Median aneurysm diameter 50–59 mm	**Migration** month—0%; 6 months—0.4%; 1 year—0.7%; >2 years—0% **Endoleak (any; type 1)** 1 month—27.3%, 2.6% 6 months—25.5%, 2.6% 1 year—22.5%, 0.4% 2 years—21.9%, 0.9% 3 years—22.1%, 1.2% 4 years—20.5%, 1.0% 5 years—16.4%, 0.8%

Device	FDA approval	Clinical study sizing	Study design	N	Follow-up	Patients excluded	Anatomical characteristics	Outcomes
Zenith	2003	Not specified (recommended 14–24% oversizing aorta and 0–20% iliacs)	Nonrandomized, prospective, multicenter clinical studies	352 (200 standard, 100 high risk, 52 roll-in)	1 month, 6 months, 1 year	• Infrarenal proximal neck length <15 mm • Infrarenal neck outer diameter <18 mm or >32 mm • Suprarenal angulation >45° or infrarenal angulation >60° • Iliac diameter <7.5 mm or >20 mm • Iliac length <10 mm • Vessel morphology not suitable for endovascular repair	• Median aneurysm diameter 50–59 mm	**Migration (>5 mm and without sequel)** 1 year—2.5%, 2.8%, 0% (standard, high risk, roll in) **Endoleak (any)** 1 year—7.4%, 8.8%, 3.4% (standard, high risk, roll in)
Powerlink	2004	10–20% relative to the neck diameter	Nonrandomized, prospective, multicenter clinical studies	192	1 month, 6 months, 1 year	• Infrarenal proximal neck length <15 mm • Infrarenal neck diameter <18 mm or >26 mm • Neck angulation >60° • Iliac artery diameter <7 mm • Iliac landing zone length <15 mm • Vessel morphology not suitable for endovascular repair	• Aneurysm diameter 51 ± 6.6 mm • Proximal seal zone length 29.3 ± 11.3 mm • Right iliac diameter 12.3 ± 2.3 mm • Left iliac diameter 12.1 ± 1.8 mm	**Migration (>5 mm without sequel)** 1 year—4.4% **Endoleak (any; new type I)** 1 month—22.7%, 0.8% 6 months—12.9%, 0% 1 year—14.1%, 0% 2 year—4.9%

	approval	sizing					characteristics	
Talent	2008	Not specified (recommended 14–24% oversizing aorta and 0–20% iliacs)	Nonrandomized, prospective, multicenter clinical studies	166	1 month, 6 months, 1 year	• Infrarenal proximal neck length of <10 mm • Infrarenal proximal neck diameter <18 mm or >32 mm • Neck angulation >60° • Iliac artery diameter of <8 mm or >22 mm • Iliac artery length of <15 mm • Vessel morphology not suitable for endovascular repair	• Aneurysm diameter 51 ± 6.6 mm • Proximal seal zone length 29.3 ± 11.3 mm • Right iliac diameter 12.3 ± 2.3 mm • Left iliac distal diameter 12.1 ± 1.8 mm	**Migration** 1 year—0.8% **Endoleak (any; type I)** 1 month—19.3%, 9.3% 1 year—9.2%, 2.5%
Endurant/ endurant II**	2010/2012	Approximately 20% greater than inner diameter	Nonrandomized, prospective, multicenter clinical studies	150	1 month, 6 months, 1 year	• Infrarenal proximal neck length <10 mm or significant calcification or thrombus • Proximal neck diameter <19 mm or >32 mm • >45° suprarenal or >60° infrarenal neck angles • Iliac fixation site diameter <8 mm or >25 mm • Aneurysmal iliac arteries or lengths <15 mm • Vessel morphology not suitable for endovascular repair	• Aneurysm diameter 55.9 ± 8.7 mm • Proximal neck length 31.0 ± 14.3 mm • Proximal neck diameter 23.5 ± 3.0 mm • Suprarenal angle 16.0 ± 10.3° • Infrarenal angle 35.2 ± 13.7° • Right iliac diameter 14.2 ± 42 mm • Left iliac diameter 13.9 ± 3.1 mm	**Migration** 1 year 0% **Endoleak (any; type I)** 1 month—16.1%, 0% 6 months—11.6%, 0% 12 months—9.8%, 0%

Modifations to the original Gore Excluder were made and tested because of aneurysm enlargement rates.

New delivery system with extended hydrophilic coating, two new limb lengths, new radiopacity on contralateral gate.

Table 2. Instructions for use—clinical studies.

5. Clinical outcomes and oversizing

The goal of EVAR is a long-term exclusion of the aneurysm, without any complications such as graft migration or endoleak. Obtaining a tight seal and adequate fixation are important in lowering intrasac pressure and limiting further disease progression. In 2009, a systematic review evaluated the relationship between oversizing and outcomes and reported that 10–20% oversizing is relatively safe and remains as the preferred sizing choice of surgeons [17].

5.1. Biomechanics and vessel remodeling

Understanding the effects of EVAR on both the vessel wall and device itself is important for making improvements in endovascular surgery. Several authors have attempted to investigate these consequences with specific consideration to the effects of oversizing. When a stent is apposed to an artery, the force created from the vessel wall opposes a stent's outward radial force. After deployment, equilibrium is achieved between the vessel and stent-graft where the radial force is proportional to the final diameter of the incorporated device [23]. Thus, radial force is significantly correlated with the degree of oversizing. If the force delivered to the vessel exceeds the equilibrium, it is plausible that the inward folding (i.e., infolding) or collapse of the graft can occur. In turn, infolding of the graft at its border can result in new interfaces between the blood flow and the graft, thus resulting in an increased risk of migration. In fact, excessive oversizing, in particular greater than 30%, has been linked to infolding of the device [24, 25]. In further analysis, Lin et al. [26] showed significantly less likelihood of folding when oversized below 23.5%. Interestingly, when stents collapse they do so asymmetrically. This has been shown in vitro where certain areas of the stent have more rigidity and thus takes on more force [23].

Another potential consequence of the radial force delivered to the vessel wall is the ability of the vessel to remodel. If the radial force is large enough, the vessel can dilate in order to accommodate for the stent graft. Several authors have reported these changes in the aneurysm neck after the EVAR [16, 27–33]. In the results of four U.S. phase II trials, neck dilatation of 3 mm or more was reported in 13–20% of patients 2 years post EVAR [30]. In a study with longer follow-up (4 years) but with smaller sample size, all patients showed at least 2 mm of neck dilatation [33]. These results follow a previous description that the self-expandable stent-grafts dilate the aortic neck until the nominal diameter of the stent graft is reached [34]. This initial adaptation has been reported for almost all the self-expandable endograft-treated aortic necks as an adjustment to the devices present and is associated with the percentage of oversizing [31]. However, it is unclear, if oversizing is associated with dilatation beyond this initial adaptation. Importantly, expansion of the aortic neck to the size of the graft is infrequently associated with adverse complications [33]. However, neck dilatation exceeding the degree of oversizing can put patients at an increased risk of developing endoleak or graft migration [35].

The mechanism, in which, a dilatation larger than the percentage of oversizing can result in migration, is thought to be through a reduction in frictional force. Thus, many authors have shown that oversizing is positively correlated with neck dilatation [25, 28, 31, 33, 36–38].

http://dx.doi.org/10.5772/66369

Conners et al. [25] reported that oversizing greater than 20% was strongly associated with an accelerated late neck expansion. However, the effect of oversizing on dilatation is not black and white. In fact, several authors have failed to find any significant correlation when compared to the postoperative diameter [27, 31, 39, 40]. For example, Cao et al. [27] failed to find an association between >15% oversizing and neck enlargement. This suggests that oversizing is not the only factor involved in the continued expansion of the aortic neck. Different endografts, stent types, and intramural or hemodynamic conditions could also play a role. It is also expected that a patient's genetics is likely to influence susceptibility to enlargement. Although unproven, the intrinsic characteristics of the host aorta could also potentially encourage remodeling. If so, markers, such as elastin and collagen may be useful preoperatively in predicting dilatation.

5.2. Graft migration

Caudal migration of the endovascular graft is one cause of the unsuccessful EVAR. In fact, migration following the EVAR has been reported in many studies with rates ranging from 0% to 45%, varying with different patient populations, follow-up times, and stent-grafts used [25, 41–43]. Migration can occur for a number of reasons, but can be best understood in the context of the biomechanical forces. If the drag force generated by the blood flow overcomes the fixation force between the endograft and aortic wall, the graft will dislodge or migrate. The main factors causing this imbalance are continued aortic neck dilatation, pulsatile blood flow acting on the seal zone, and mechanical or biological features complicating the attachment. Continuous exposure of displacement forces in the direction perpendicular to the endograft may cause eccentric graft compression and result in migration [44]. In turn, graft migration can lead to other complications, such as, endoleak, occlusion, or rupture. In addition, displacement of the stent graft from its apposition site may result in the need for secondary intervention. Since graft oversizing has been linked to aortic dilatation and because it plays an important part in achieving adequate fixation, correctly oversizing the device can potentially limit migration.

Several studies have investigated the association between oversizing and device migration [25, 27, 31, 33, 40, 45–49]. It should be noted that the definition of migration may vary from study to study and the amount of migration can ultimately be associated with worse outcomes. For example, migration of a few millimeters, when compared to complete migration into the aneurysm sac, will have significantly different consequences. Oversizing can help limit migration by increasing the contact pressure between the vessel wall and device [50]. One experimental study found that when oversized an average of 27.7%, 336 g was needed to cause migration, as opposed to only 305 g needed to displace grafts oversized an average of 14.4% [15]. In terms of specific ranges, oversizing >20% seems to require a greater pullout force than when sized under 20% [15]. This result can help explain the trend toward greater oversizing in patients experiencing migration when oversized a mean of 23.5% vs. 18.2% [25]. In a larger study of 1082 patients, oversizing 10–30% had the lowest percentage of migration [46]. Not oversizing enough, e.g., 10% will require lower magnitudes necessary to cause migration compared to devices oversized 20% [51]. Interestingly, migration has been suggested to occur after two displacement forces, one to start the movement and the second, substantially greater, force to cause significant caudal movement [51].

As a potential solution for migration, several devices are now made with active fixation (barbs, anchors, and pins). Barbs and hooks increase the force needed to dislodge a graft [52]. Yet, migration of these grafts can still occur. Thus, when considering the connection of oversizing and device migration, the device type may play a crucial role. Increasing data has indicated that the biomechanical forces vary between devices with regard to active fixation. Kratzberg et al. [48] has shown that as the number of barbs penetrating the aortic wall increases, so does the pullout force. However, the displacement force is not significantly affected by oversizing until above 30%, at which less force is then needed to dislodge the graft [48, 51]. Importantly, grafts oversized >30% can experience significant circumferential deformation/folding at its perimeter that negatively affects the attachment [48]. This has been suggested as a major reason for the lower pullout force for grafts oversized >30% compared to those sized 4–10%, 11–20%, and 21–30% [48]. Sternbergh et al. [40] had similar findings, where they found a 14 time increase in device migration of 5 mm or more for zenith (active fixation) stent-grafts oversized above 30%. Thus, excessive oversizing of aortic stent-grafts with active fixation may come with adverse outcomes. Congruently, Vad et al. have proposed sizing these stents up to 15% [50].

5.3. Endoleak

Although the pathogenesis of aneurysm enlargement is not completely understood, it is generally accepted that the persistent blood flow into the aneurysm sac can lead to further expansion and potentially rupture. Thus, incomplete exclusion and resulting perigraft flow, termed as endoleak, is a significant complication of EVAR. In particular, type I (incomplete seal) and III (mechanical failure of the graft) endoleaks are associated with worse outcomes, with type 1A (proximal) leak posing the greatest risk of rupture [14]. Endoleak is amongst the most common failures reported with rates ranging from approximately 5 to 40% [14, 53–55]. Furthermore, some authors estimate that endoleaks account for over 60% of EVAR reinterventions [56]. Importantly, type I leaks have been attributed to inadequate sizing of endografts [14]. Thus, the impact of oversizing and its role in limiting endoleaks has received considerable attention.

One mechanism in which oversizing has been suggested to cause endoleak is through infolding of the endograft. As mentioned earlier, higher degrees of oversizing have been linked to greater folds [24]. This is significant because the presence of endoleak was subsequently correlated to the size of the biggest fold [24]. Another cause of endoleak is due to the expansion of the aorta often seen from excessive oversizing. Aortic dilatation can create gaps between the endograft and vessel wall, thus allowing the blood to flow into the aneurysm. A third mechanism for endoleaks is from undersizing the aortic stent graft. Undersized grafts exert a weaker radial force on the vessel wall and thus can be influenced by smaller displacement forces from the pulsatile blood flow. In turn, a decrease in radial force can lead to the development of proximal endoleaks [57]. This is likely to occur through the spaces that exist between the stent graft and vessel wall. In particular, separation during the decreasing phase of hydrostatic pressure has been described [57]. This suggests a delayed deformation as the pressure on the attachment site decreases and the aorta relaxes.

Many studies have investigated endoleaks, but few have looked at the relationship between leak and oversizing. One such study of 2146 patients undergoing EVAR with multiple device types, showed a decreased risk of proximal endoleak starting at 10% oversizing with narrow confidence intervals up to 25% [14]. In another study, oversizing >20% was associated with fewer endoleaks (all) and less aneurysm sac enlargement, with the lowest rate of endoleaks occurring between 20 and 25% [58]. A mechanics study had similar findings suggesting that oversizing 20% helps prevent the occurrence of type I endoleaks [57].

Still, several studies failed to find any significance between oversizing and endoleaks, including one that investigated those oversized >30% [40, 54, 59, 60]. Several of these studies were difficult to interpret, due to varying population characteristics and methodology. One reason for this is that oversizing can be complicated by several factors, one being the conditions at the attachment sites. Atherosclerotic plaque, thrombus, and calcifications can interfere with the device-wall interface. Intuitively, the presence of plaque between the graft and the vessel lowers the frictional coefficient, and thus the force too. Amblard et al. suggested that the plaque configuration at the attachment site can be used to predict type I endoleaks [57]. Apposition site morphology has also been thought to contribute to the risk of endoleak. Conical necks, in particular, can pose increased risk because oversizing in the proximal and distal portions of these necks are uneven. This often results in one end being undersized. Thus, greater oversizing may be appropriate if the characteristics are difficult, such as, a reverse tapered neck [61].

6. Histology of the attachment sites and oversizing

Several adaptations occur to the arterial wall after EVAR. Few studies have looked at the effects of oversizing in the abdominal aorta, but the changes seen in the thoracic aorta can still provide valuable information. When a stent graft is implanted, a foreign body reaction can result. One adaptation is a considerable loss of elasticity, especially at the area of compression, regardless of the percentage of oversizing [62]. The same study showed that the max strength sustained and the stress supported by fragments of the aortic wall suffered a linear and progressive loss with increased oversizing [62]. This change can be contributed to a reorganization and change in quantity of collagen and elastic fibers distributed around the apposition sites. In particular, collagen increases in the aortic wall irrespective of the degree of oversizing [62] On the other hand, the amount of muscle fibers decrease in the inner third of the wall with more oversizing [62]. Importantly, oversizing >40% showed evidence of disruption of the fiber content and formation of an aneurysm within the aortic wall [63]. These results should be taken with caution, as the biology of the vessel at the infrarenal level may differ.

7. Imaging/preoperative measurements

Accurate sizing of aortic stent-grafts depends on precise preoperative measurements of the aorta and iliac arteries. In the past, measurements were done using computerized tomography angiography (CTA) axial images, but more recently three-dimensional (3D) reconstructions with center lumen line (CLL) analysis have taken over [64, 65]. The use of CLL has improved the measurement of preoperative diameters and lengths with superior outcomes, and less intra- and interobserver variability [64, 66]. Yet, accurate and reproducible measurement remains a challenge. Arteries are frequently not perfect circles and thus measurement can vary based on the axis. In response, some have proposed alternative methods that are yet to be validated, such as using circumference [67]. Thus, while using CLL, it is important to follow the manufacturer's IFU measurement instructions. This has become even more evident, as an increasing number of patients undergoing EVAR today have complex apposition site features complicating their measurement.

The use of dynamic CTA can also provide some valuable insight for preoperative planning. Using dynamic CTA, several authors have found that the aortic and iliac arteries diameter, circumference, angles, and lengths change during the cardiac cycle [68–70]. Specifically, an asymmetrical distension is seen with smaller dimensions occurring during diastole. Interestingly, preoperative aneurysm neck pulsatility remains similar even years after EVAR, but the baseline pulsatility is higher for those who experience graft migration [71]. Furthermore, distension due to dynamic changes in the iliac arteries has been suggested to be a cause of distal endoleak [68]. These two observations show how the pulsatility of a patient's vessels can contribute to the over or undersizing of stent-grafts and ultimately lead to poor outcomes. In fact, in one study, endografts were inadequately sized for approximately 25% of patients [72]. Since pulsatility can vary from patient to patient, measurement of those with complex vessel dynamics should be given appropriate attention. Additionally, the fact that vessels expand asymmetrically further supports the use of oversizing as a way to limit gaps between the graft and vessel wall. To account for these dynamic changes during the cardiac cycle, oversizing as much as 20% has been recommended [17, 68].

8. Recent sizing, our experience, conclusions

Advancements in endovascular technique, imaging technology, and device design have led to an expanded use of EVAR in the treatment of AAAs.

Aortic stent-grafts create a new channel for the blood flow and thus shield the diseased aortic wall from continued pressure. A number of factors influence the sealing and fixation of self-expandable stent-grafts. Some include: (1) vessel shape/diameter, (2) seal zone length, (3) angulation/tortuosity, (4) calcification/thrombus, (5) device design (active fixation, material), and (6) vessel hemodynamics. Thus, the anatomy and conditions at or around the apposition sites are important to consider when sizing.

Some recent studies have provided the degree of oversizing of their cohorts and reported outcomes. The ENGAGE study of 1262 patients (approximately one-fifth outside IFU) oversized 20% with respect to the inner vessel diameter reported with no stent migration at 1 year and with satisfactory outcomes [42]. Pitton et al. showed strong results after 10-year follow-up with 20–25% oversizing of proximal diameters and 10–15% oversizing distally [73]. Similarly, in a recent study, 351 patients (mean outer-to-outer wall oversizing 17.7 ± 10.7%) from 2003 to 2014 showed that >20% oversizing was associated with decreased rates of endoleaks (all) compared with 10–20% oversizing, with the lowest rates in patients oversized 20–25% [58]. Interestingly, larger infrarenal neck diameters were associated with less oversizing. This is suggestive that larger vessels are at risk of being undersized. Although the rate of limb occlusion after EVAR is relatively low, it is worth mentioning that greater than 15% oversizing at the iliac artery was identified as an independent risk factor for limb occlusion [74].

Almost all the recommendations for the degree of oversizing made by manufacturers are based on the patients with ideal conditions, such as, straight aortic necks and nontortuous iliac arteries. This can be problematic when endografts are delivered to complicated apposition sites. For consistency in preoperative measurement, surgeons should follow the protocols outlined by each device manufacturer, as to which axis measurements should be taken from. With regards to oversizing, sizing up to 25% in the aortic neck appears to increase the radial force and lower the risk of proximal endoleak. Although inconclusive, additional oversizing above 25% may be associated with greater risk of aortic dilatation or graft infolding with the potential to cause migration. Ultimately, oversizing, using the current standard of 10–20% remains safe and effective. As more complicated EVAR patients present, practice may need to be adjusted on a patient-specific basis.

Author details

Alex Sher and Rami O. Tadros*

Address all correspondence to: rami.tadros@mountsinai.org

The Mount Sinai Medical Center, New York, NY, USA

References

[1] Ho, P., W.K. Yiu, G.C.Y. Cheung, S.W.K. Cheng, A.C.W. Ting, and J.T.C. Poon, *Systematic review of clinical trials comparing open and endovascular treatment of abdominal aortic aneurysm*. Surg Pract, 2006. **10**(1): 24–37.

[2] Reilly, L.M., *Pro: endovascular repair of abdominal aortic aneurysms reduces perioperative morbidity and mortality*. J Cardiothorac Vasc Anesth, 2003. **17**(5): 655–8.

[3] Blankensteijn, J.D., S.E. de Jong, M. Prinssen, A.C. van der Ham, J. Buth, S.M. van Sterkenburg, H.J. Verhagen, E. Buskens, and D.E. Grobbee, *Two-year outcomes after conventional or endovascular repair of abdominal aortic aneurysms*. N Engl J Med, 2005. **352**(23): 2398–405.

[4] Greenhalgh, R. M. Brown, L. C. Epstein, D. Kwong, G. P. S. Powell, J. T. Sculpher, M. J. Thompson, S. G. EVAR Trial Participants*Endovascular aneurysm repair versus open repair in patients with abdominal aortic aneurysm (EVAR trial 1): randomised controlled trial*. Lancet, 2005. **365**(9478): 2179–86.

[5] Greenhalgh, R.M., L.C. Brown, J.T. Powell, S.G. Thompson, D. Epstein, and M.J. Sculpher, *Endovascular versus open repair of abdominal aortic aneurysm.* N Engl J Med, 2010. **362**(20): 1863–71.

[6] Schermerhorn, M.L., A.J. O'Malley, A. Jhaveri, P. Cotterill, F. Pomposelli, and B.E. Landon, *Endovascular vs. open repair of abdominal aortic aneurysms in the Medicare population.* N Engl J Med, 2008. **358**(5): 464–74.

[7] Veith, F.J., R.A. Baum, T. Ohki, M. Amor, M. Adiseshiah, J.D. Blankensteijn, J. Buth, T.A. Chuter, R.M. Fairman, G. Gilling-Smith, P.L. Harris, K.J. Hodgson, B.R. Hopkinson, K. Ivancev, B.T. Katzen, M. Lawrence-Brown, G.H. Meier, M. Malina, M.S. Makaroun, J.C. Parodi, G.M. Richter, G.D. Rubin, W.J. Stelter, G.H. White, R.A. White, W. Wisselink, and C.K. Zarins, *Nature and significance of endoleaks and endotension: summary of opinions expressed at an international conference.* J Vasc Surg, 2002. **35**(5): 1029–35.

[8] Hellinger, J.C., *Endovascular repair of thoracic and abdominal aortic aneurysms: pre- and post-procedural imaging.* Tech Vasc Interv Radiol, 2005. **8**(1): 2–15.

[9] Parodi, J.C., J.C. Palmaz, and H.D. Barone, *Transfemoral intraluminal graft implantation for abdominal aortic aneurysms.* Ann Vasc Surg, 1991. **5**(6): 491–9.

[10] Balko, A., G.J. Piasecki, D.M. Shah, W.I. Carney, R.W. Hopkins, and B.T. Jackson, *Transfemoral placement of intraluminal polyurethane prosthesis for abdominal aortic aneurysm.* J Surg Res, 1986. **40**(4): 305–9.

[11] Lawrence, D.D., Jr., C. Charnsangavej, K.C. Wright, C. Gianturco, and S. Wallace, *Percutaneous endovascular graft: experimental evaluation.* Radiology, 1987. **163**(2): 357–60.

[12] Mirich, D., K.C. Wright, S. Wallace, T. Yoshioka, D.D. Lawrence, Jr., C. Charnsangavej, and C. Gianturco, *Percutaneously placed endovascular grafts for aortic aneurysms: feasibility study.* Radiology, 1989. **170**(3 Pt 2): 1033–7.

[13] Laborde, J.C., J.C. Parodi, M.F. Clem, F.O. Tio, H.D. Barone, F.J. Rivera, C.E. Encarnacion, and J.C. Palmaz, *Intraluminal bypass of abdominal aortic aneurysm: feasibility study.* Radiology, 1992. **184**(1): 185–90.

[14] Mohan, I.V., R.J. Laheij, and P.L. Harris, *Risk factors for endoleak and the evidence for stent-graft oversizing in patients undergoing endovascular aneurysm repair.* Eur J Vasc Endovasc Surg, 2001. **21**(4): 344–9.

[15] Lambert, A.W., D.J. Williams, J.S. Budd, and M. Horrocks, *Experimental assessment of proximal stent-graft (intervascular) fixation in human cadaveric infrarenal aortas.* Eur J Vasc Endovasc Surg, 1999. **17**(1): 60–5.

[16] Rodway, A.D., J.T. Powell, L.C. Brown, and R.M. Greenhalgh, *Do abdominal aortic aneurysm necks increase in size faster after endovascular than open repair?* Eur J Vasc Endovasc Surg, 2008. **35**(6): 685–93.

[17] van Prehn, J., F.J. Schlosser, B.E. Muhs, H.J. Verhagen, F.L. Moll, and J.A. van Herwaarden, *Oversizing of aortic stent grafts for abdominal aneurysm repair: a systematic review of the benefits and risks.* Eur J Vasc Endovasc Surg, 2009. **38**(1): 42–53.

[18] Matsumae, M., H. Uchida, and S. Teramoto, *An experimental study of a new sutureless intraluminal graft with an elastic ring that can attach itself to the vessel wall. A preliminary report*. J Vasc Surg, 1988. **8**(1): 38–44.

[19] Dotter, C.T., R.W. Buschmann, M.K. McKinney, and J. Rosch, *Transluminal expandable nitinol coil stent grafting: preliminary report*. Radiology, 1983. **147**(1): 259–60.

[20] Cragg, A.H., G. Lund, J.A. Rysavy, E. Salomonowitz, W.R. Castaneda-Zuniga, and K. Amplatz, *Percutaneous arterial grafting*. Radiology, 1984. **150**(1): 45–9.

[21] Moritz, J.D., S. Rotermund, D.P. Keating, and J.W. Oestmann, *Infrarenal abdominal aortic aneurysms: implications of CT evaluation of size and configuration for placement of endovascular aortic grafts*. Radiology, 1996. **198**(2): 463–6.

[22] Armon, M.P., S.W. Yusuf, S.C. Whitaker, R.H. Gregson, P.W. Wenham, and B.R. Hopkinson, *The anatomy of abdominal aortic aneurysms: implications for sizing of endovascular grafts*. Eur J Vasc Endovasc Surg, 1997. **13**(4): 398–402.

[23] Johnston, C.R., K. Lee, J. Flewitt, R. Moore, G.M. Dobson, and G.M. Thornton, *The mechanical properties of endovascular stents: an in vitro assessment*. Cardiovasc Eng, 2010. **10**(3): 128–35.

[24] Schurink, G.W., N.J. Aarts, J.M. van Baalen, L.J. Schultze Kool, and J.H. van Bockel, *Stent attachment site-related endoleakage after stent graft treatment: an in vitro study of the effects of graft size, stent type, and atherosclerotic wall changes*. J Vasc Surg, 1999. **30**(4): 658–67.

[25] Conners, M.S., 3rd, W.C. Sternbergh, 3rd, G. Carter, B.H. Tonnessen, M. Yoselevitz, and S.R. Money, *Endograft migration one to four years after endovascular abdominal aortic aneurysm repair with the AneuRx device: a cautionary note*. J Vasc Surg, 2002. **36**(3): 476–84.

[26] Lin, K.K., J.A. Kratzberg, and M.L. Raghavan, *Role of aortic stent graft oversizing and barb characteristics on folding*. J Vasc Surg, 2012. **55**(5): 1401–9.

[27] Cao, P., F. Verzini, G. Parlani, P.D. Rango, B. Parente, G. Giordano, S. Mosca, and A. Maselli, *Predictive factors and clinical consequences of proximal aortic neck dilatation in 230 patients undergoing abdominal aorta aneurysm repair with self-expandable stent-grafts*. J Vasc Surg, 2003. **37**(6): 1200–5.

[28] Badran, M.F., D.A. Gould, I. Raza, R.G. McWilliams, O. Brown, P.L. Harris, G.L. Gilling-Smith, J. Brennan, D. White, S. Meakin, and P.C. Rowlands, *Aneurysm neck diameter after endovascular repair of abdominal aortic aneurysms*. J Vasc Interv Radiol, 2002. **13**(9 Pt 1): 887–92.

[29] Napoli, V., S.G. Sardella, I. Bargellini, P. Petruzzi, R. Cioni, C. Vignali, M. Ferrari, and C. Bartolozzi, *Evaluation of the proximal aortic neck enlargement following endovascular repair of abdominal aortic aneurysm: 3-years experience*. Eur Radiol, 2003. **13**(8): 1962–71.

[30] Dillavou, E.D., S. Muluk, and M.S. Makaroun, *Is neck dilatation after endovascular aneurysm repair graft dependent? Results of 4 US Phase II trials*. Vasc Endovascular Surg, 2005. **39**(1): 47–54.

[31] Sampaio, S.M., J.M. Panneton, G. Mozes, J.C. Andrews, A.A. Noel, M. Kalra, T.C. Bower, K.J. Cherry, T.M. Sullivan, and P. Gloviczki, *Aortic neck dilation after endovascular abdominal aortic aneurysm repair: should oversizing be blamed?* Ann Vasc Surg, 2006. **20**(3): 338–45.

[32] Diehm, N., F. Dick, B.T. Katzen, J. Schmidli, C. Kalka, and I. Baumgartner, *Aortic neck dilatation after endovascular abdominal aortic aneurysm repair: a word of caution.* J Vasc Surg, 2008. **47**(4): 886–92.

[33] Monahan, T.S., T.A. Chuter, L.M. Reilly, J.H. Rapp, and J.S. Hiramoto, *Long-term follow-up of neck expansion after endovascular aortic aneurysm repair.* J Vasc Surg, 2010. **52**(2): 303–7.

[34] Grenacher, L., S. Rohde, E. Ganger, J. Deutsch, G.W. Kauffmann, and G.M. Richter, *In vitro comparison of self-expanding versus balloon-expandable stents in a human ex vivo model.* Cardiovasc Intervent Radiol, 2006. **29**(2): 249–54.

[35] Oliveira, N.G., F.B. Goncalves, M.J. Van Rijn, F. Moll, S.T. Raa, S. Hoeks, J. Hendriks, and H. Verhagen, *Neck dilatation after endovascular aneurysm repair rarely exceeds the implanted endograft on long-term follow-up.* J Vasc Surg, June 2016. **63**(6), supplement, 20S-21S.

[36] Zhang, J., W. Guo, X.P. Liu, T. Yin, and X. Jia, *The dilatation of the proximal neck after endovascular repair of abdominal aortic aneurysm.* Zhonghua Wai Ke Za Zhi, 2011. **49**(5): 392–5.

[37] Prinssen, M., J.J. Wever, W.P. Mali, B.C. Eikelboom, and J.D. Blankensteijn, *Concerns for the durability of the proximal abdominal aortic aneurysm endograft fixation from a 2-year and 3-year longitudinal computed tomography angiography study.* J Vasc Surg, 2001. **33**(2 Suppl): S64–9.

[38] Makaroun, M.S. and D.H. Deaton, *Is proximal aortic neck dilatation after endovascular aneurysm exclusion a cause for concern?* J Vasc Surg, 2001. **33**(2 Suppl): S39–45.

[39] Wever, J.J., A.J. de Nie, J.D. Blankensteijn, I.A. Broeders, W.P. Mali, and B.C. Eikelboom, *Dilatation of the proximal neck of infrarenal aortic aneurysms after endovascular AAA repair.* Eur J Vasc Endovasc Surg, 2000. **19**(2): 197–201.

[40] Sternbergh, W.C., 3rd, Money, S.R., Greenberg, R.K., and Chuter, T.A., *Influence of endograft oversizing on device migration, endoleak, aneurysm shrinkage, and aortic neck dilation: results from the Zenith multicenter trial.* J Vasc Surg, 2004. **39**(1): 20–6.

[41] Resch, T., K. Ivancev, J. Brunkwall, U. Nyman, M. Malina, and B. Lindblad, *Distal migration of stent-grafts after endovascular repair of abdominal aortic aneurysms.* J Vasc Interv Radiol, 1999. **10**(3): 257–64; discussion 265–6.

[42] Stokmans, R.A., J.A. Teijink, T.L. Forbes, D. Bockler, P.J. Peeters, V. Riambau, P.D. Hayes, and M.R. van Sambeek, *Early results from the ENGAGE registry: real-world performance of the endurant stent graft for endovascular AAA repair in 1262 patients.* Eur J Vasc Endovasc Surg, 2012. **44**(4): 369–75.

[43] England, A., J.S. Butterfield, N. Jones, C.N. McCollum, A. Nasim, M. Welch, and R.J. Ashleigh, *Device migration after endovascular abdominal aortic aneurysm repair: experience with a talent stent-graft.* J Vasc Interv Radiol, 2004. **15**(12): 1399–405.

[44] Wolf, Y.G., B.B. Hill, W.A. Lee, C.M. Corcoran, T.J. Fogarty, and C.K. Zarins, *Eccentric stent graft compression: an indicator of insecure proximal fixation of aortic stent graft.* J Vasc Surg, 2001. **33**(3): 481–7.

[45] Mohan, I.V., P.L. Harris, C.J. Van Marrewijk, R.J. Laheij, and T.V. How, *Factors and forces influencing stent-graft migration after endovascular aortic aneurysm repair*. J Endovasc Ther, 2002. **9**(6): 748–55.

[46] Zarins, C.K., D.A. Bloch, T. Crabtree, A.H. Matsumoto, R.A. White, and T.J. Fogarty, *Stent graft migration after endovascular aneurysm repair: importance of proximal fixation*. J Vasc Surg, 2003. **38**(6): 1264–72; discussion 1272.

[47] Oberhuber, A., A. Schwarz, M.H. Hoffmann, O. Klass, K.H. Orend, and B. Muhling, *Influence of different self-expanding stent-graft types on remodeling of the aortic neck after endovascular aneurysm repair*. J Endovasc Ther, 2010. **17**(6): 677–84.

[48] Kratzberg, J.A., J. Golzarian, and M.L. Raghavan, *Role of graft oversizing in the fixation strength of barbed endovascular grafts*. J Vasc Surg, 2009. **49**(6): 1543–53.

[49] Koncar, I., D. Krsmanovic, V. Isailovic, L. Davidovic, and N. Filipovic, *Computer simulation of endoluminal stent-graft migration*. Int J Artif Organs, 2012. **35** (8): 556.

[50] Vad, S., A. Eskinazi, T. Corbett, T. McGloughlin, and J.P. Vande Geest, *Determination of coefficient of friction for self-expanding stent-grafts*. J Biomech Eng, 2010. **132**(12): 121007.

[51] Zhou, S.S., T.V. How, S. Rao Vallabhaneni, G.L. Gilling-Smith, J.A. Brennan, P.L. Harris, and R. McWilliams, *Comparison of the fixation strength of standard and fenestrated stent-grafts for endovascular abdominal aortic aneurysm repair*. J Endovasc Ther, 2007. **14**(2): 168–75.

[52] Malina, M., B. Lindblad, K. Ivancev, M. Lindh, J. Malina, and J. Brunkwall, *Endovascular AAA exclusion: will stents with hooks and barbs prevent stent-graft migration?* J Endovasc Surg, 1998. **5**(4): 310–7.

[53] Kaladji, A., E. Steintmetz, Y. Goueffic, M. Bartoli, and A. Cardon, *Long-term results of large stent grafts to treat abdominal aortic aneurysms*. Ann Vasc Surg, 2015. **29**(7): 1416–25.

[54] Petrik, P.V. and W.S. Moore, *Endoleaks following endovascular repair of abdominal aortic aneurysm: the predictive value of preoperative anatomic factors—a review of 100 cases*. J Vasc Surg, 2001. **33**(4): 739–44.

[55] Lal, B.K., W. Zhou, Z. Li, T. Kyriakides, J. Matsumura, F.A. Lederle, and J. Freischlag, *Predictors and outcomes of endoleaks in the veterans affairs open versus endovascular repair (OVER) trial of abdominal aortic Aneurysms*. J Vasc Surg, 2015. **62**(6): 1394–404.

[56] Al-Jubouri, M., A.J. Comerota, S. Thakur, F. Aziz, S. Wanjiku, D. Paolini, J.P. Pigott, and F. Lurie, *Reintervention after EVAR and open surgical repair of AAA: a 15-year experience*. Ann Surg, 2013. **258**(4): 652–7; discussion 657–8.

[57] Amblard, A., H.W. Berre, B. Bou-Said, and M. Brunet, *Analysis of type I endoleaks in a stented abdominal aortic aneurysm*. Med Eng Phys, 2009. **31**(1): 27–33.

[58] Beckerman, W.E., R.O. Tadros, A. Sher, J.R. Power, C.Y.M. Png, M. Tardiff, M.L. Marin, and P.L. Faries, *Influence of infrarenal oversizing of aortic stent grafts on patient outcomes*. J Vasc Surg, June 2016. **63**(6); supplement, 164S.

[59] Sampaio, S.M., J.M. Panneton, G.I. Mozes, J.C. Andrews, T.C. Bower, M. Karla, A.A. Noel, K.J. Cherry, T. Sullivan, and P. Gloviczki, *Proximal type I endoleak after endovascular abdominal aortic aneurysm repair: predictive factors*. Ann Vasc Surg, 2004. **18**(6): 621–8.

[60] Matsumura, J.S. and W.S. Moore, *Clinical consequences of periprosthetic leak after endovascular repair of abdominal aortic aneurysm. Endovascular technologies investigators*. J Vasc Surg, 1998. **27**(4): 606–13.

[61] Mwipatayi, B.P., A. Picardo, J. Wong, S.D. Thomas, and V. Vijayan, *Endovascular repair of abdominal aortic aneurysms with reverse taper neck anatomy using the Endurant stent-graft: analysis of stent-graft oversizing*. J Endovasc Ther, 2013. **20**(4): 514–22.

[62] Sincos, I.R., R. Aun, E.S. da Silva, S. Belczak, M. de Lourdes Higuchi, V.C. Gornati, P.N. Gigglio, A.P. Baptista, and L.F. de Figueiredo, *Impact of stent-graft oversizing on the thoracic aorta: experimental study in a porcine model*. J Endovasc Ther, 2011. **18**(4): 576–84.

[63] Sincos, I.R., E.S. da Silva, S.Q. Belczak, A.P. Baptista Sincos, M. de Lourdes Higuchi, V. Gornati, J.P. Otoch, and R. Aun, *Histologic analysis of stent graft oversizing in the thoracic aorta*. J Vasc Surg, 2013. **58**(6): 1644–1651.e4.

[64] Sobocinski, J., H. Chenorhokian, B. Maurel, M. Midulla, A. Hertault, M. Le Roux, R. Azzaoui, and S. Haulon, *The benefits of EVAR planning using a 3D workstation*. Eur J Vasc Endovasc Surg, 2013. **46**(4): 418–23.

[65] Kaladji, A., A. Lucas, G. Kervio, P. Haigron, and A. Cardon, *Sizing for endovascular aneurysm repair: clinical evaluation of a new automated three-dimensional software*. Ann Vasc Surg, 2010. **24**(7): 912–20.

[66] de Vries, J.P., *The proximal neck: the remaining barrier to a complete EVAR world*. Semin Vasc Surg, 2012. **25**(4): 182–6.

[67] Tielliu, I.F., R.V. Buijs, M.J. Greuter, T. Vainas, Wallis de Vries, B.M., Prins, T.R., and C.J. Zeebregts, *Circumference as an alternative for diameter measurement in endovascular aneurysm repair*. Med Hypotheses, 2015. **85**(2): 230–3.

[68] Pol, J.A., M. Truijers, J.A. van der Vliet, M.F. Fillinger, S.P. Marra, W.K. Renema, L.J. Oostveen, L.J. Kool, and J.D. Blankensteijn, *Impact of dynamic computed tomographic angiography on endograft sizing for endovascular aneurysm repair*. J Endovasc Ther, 2009. **16**(5): 546–51.

[69] van Keulen, J.W., J. van Prehn, M. Prokop, F.L. Moll, and J.A. van Herwaarden, *Dynamics of the aorta before and after endovascular aneurysm repair: a systematic review*. Eur J Vasc Endovasc Surg, 2009. **38**(5): 586–96.

[70] Teutelink, A., A. Rutten, B.E. Muhs, M. Olree, J.A. van Herwaarden, A.M. de Vos, M. Prokop, F.L. Moll, and H.J. Verhagen, *Pilot study of dynamic cine CT angiography for the evaluation of abdominal aortic aneurysms: implications for endograft treatment*. J Endovasc Ther, 2006. **13**(2): 139–44.

http://dx.doi.org/10.5772/66369

[71] van Keulen, J.W., F.L. Moll, G.K. Barwegen, E.P. Vonken, and J.A. van Herwaarden, *Pulsatile distension of the proximal aneurysm neck is larger in patients with stent graft migration.* Eur J Vasc Endovasc Surg, 2010. **40**(3): 326–31.

[72] Iezzi, R., C. Di Stasi, F. Pirro, R. Dattesi, F. Snider, and L. Bonomo, *Dynamic cine CT-angiography (CTA) of the proximal aneurysm neck: conformational changes during the cardiac cycle with possible consequences for endograft selection and sizing.* Cardiovasc Intervent Radiol, 2010. **33**: 170.

[73] Pitton, M.B., T. Scheschkowski, M. Ring, S. Herber, K. Oberholzer, A. Leicher-Duber, A. Neufang, W. Schmiedt, and C. Duber, *Ten-year follow-up of endovascular aneurysm treatment with talent stent-grafts.* Cardiovasc Intervent Radiol, 2009. **32**(5): 906–17.

[74] Mantas, G.K., C.N. Antonopoulos, G.S. Sfyroeras, K.G. Moulakakis, J.D. Kakisis, S.N. Mylonas, and C.D. Liapis, *Factors predisposing to endograft limb occlusion after endovascular aortic repair.* Eur J Vasc Endovasc Surg, 2015. **49**(1): 39–44.

Chapter 8

Coexistence of the Aortic Aneurysm with the Main Vein Anomalies: Its Potential Clinical Implications and Vascular Complication

Michał Polguj, Katarzyna Stefańczyk and
Ludomir Stefańczyk

Additional information is available at the end of the chapter

http://dx.doi.org/10.5772/66768

Abstract

Four major variations of the venous system in the retroperitoneal space are the retroaortic left renal vein, left renal vein collar, left-sided inferior vena cava, and caval duplication. During surgery, especially, injury in veins is responsible for the most unexpected intraoperative bleeding. Therefore, above-mentioned anomalies pose potential hazards to surgeons during treatment of abdominal aortic aneurysm. Preoperative diagnosis is highly desirable but is not always available so, during abdominal surgery, familiarity with the anatomy of the most common types of venous variations is the first step toward preventing vascular injury. The chapter includes information describing the demographic, clinical, and morphological characteristics of the presence of the aforementioned main vein anomalies including: gender distribution, frequency in population, the most commonly reported symptoms, and associate complications. Massive intraoperative bleeding may be dangerous during aortic dissection; however, venous bleeding is more complicated than arterial hemorrhage. Significant venous bleeding, in particular, can occur if major retroperitoneal venous anomalies are present. The anomalous veins are typically thin-walled, dilated, and tortuous. As a result, manipulation of these veins during abdominal aortic surgery places the patient at high risk of long-term massive hemorrhage.

Keywords: aortic aneurysm, vascular variations, retroaortic left renal vein, left renal vein collar, left-sided inferior vena cava, caval duplication

1. Introduction

There are four major variations of the venous system in the retroperitoneal space: retroaortic left renal vein, left renal vein collar, left-sided inferior vena cava, and caval duplication [1, 2] (**Figures 1–3**). These anomalies pose potential hazards to surgeons during treatment of abdominal aortic aneurysm. An injury to an unrecognized anomalous vessels can result in severe hemorrhage [3, 4]. Especially, injury to veins is responsible for the most unexpected intraoperative bleeding [4, 5]. The anomalous veins are typically thin-walled, dilated, and tortuous [6], and manipulation of these veins during abdominal aortic surgery places the patient at high risk of massive hemorrhage [1, 7]. The majority of cases of retroaortic left renal vein, left renal vein collar, left-sided inferior vena cava, and caval duplication are diagnosed incidentally on the base of radiological examinations performed for other reasons, but these variations can have significant clinical implications [1, 5].

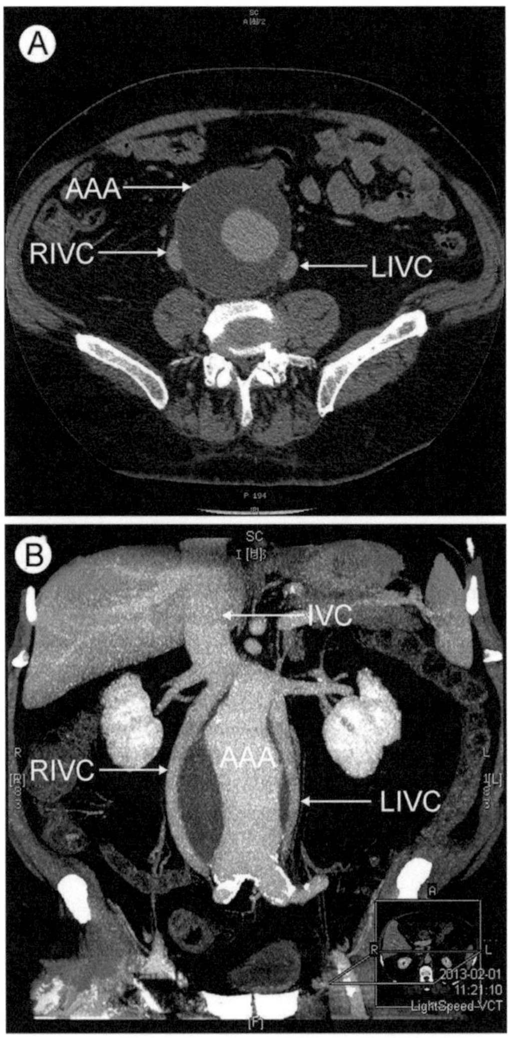

Figure 1. Computed tomography investigation of the abdomen with duplication of the inferior vena cava (CT-64-row MDCT scanner, Light-speed VCT, GE, Waukesha, Wisconsin, USA). (A) Transverse scan on L3 level, (B) three-dimensional computed tomography reconstruction of the vessels (posterior view). Ao: aorta, AAA: abdominal aortic aneurysm, IVC: inferior vena cava, LIVC: left inferior vena cava, RIVC: right inferior vena cava.

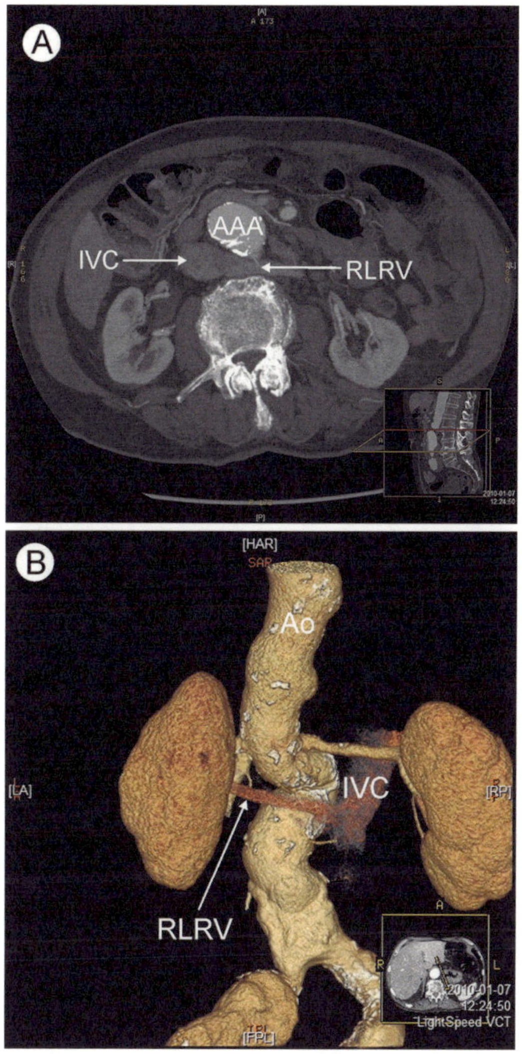

Figure 2. Computed tomography investigation of the abdomen with retroaortic left renal vein (CT-64-row MDCT scanner, Light-speed VCT, GE, Waukesha, Wisconsin, USA). (A) Transverse scan on L2 level, (B) three-dimensional computed tomography reconstruction of the vessels (posterior view). Ao: aorta, AAA: abdominal aortic aneurysm, IVC: inferior vena cava, RLRV: retroaortic left renal vein.

Preoperative diagnosis is highly desirable but not always available and most venous anomalies are diagnosed during operations. Therefore, during abdominal surgery, familiarity with the anatomy of the most common types of venous variations is the first step toward preventing vascular injury [5].

Additionally, compression of surrounding vessels by abdominal aortic aneurysm or atherosclerotic aorta forms a rich collateral circulation that exists in the abdomen and prevents the presence of ischemic symptoms [8, 9]. However, when hemodynamic compensation mechanisms begin to fail, the effects may be extremely serious. Such coexistence may complicate surgical treatment and thus predispose the patient to thrombosis [10–12].

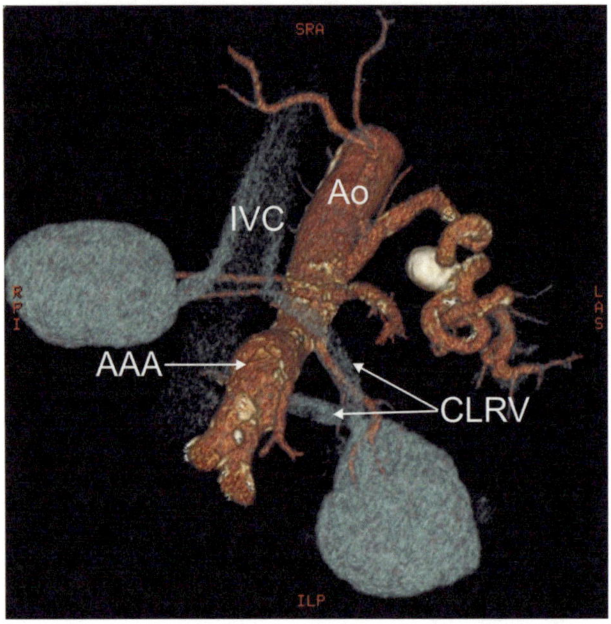

Figure 3. Three-dimensional computed tomography reconstruction of the vessels (CT-64-row MDCT scanner, Lightspeed VCT, GE, Waukesha, Wisconsin, USA). Ao: aorta, AAA: abdominal aortic aneurysm, CLRV: circumaortic left renal vein, IVC: inferior vena cava.

2. Duplication of the inferior vena cava

Duplication of the inferior vena cava is defined as an anomaly with two large veins situated on both sides of the abdominal aorta (**Figure 1**). These veins usually join to form one vein at the level of the origin of the renal arteries [1, 2]. It is a rare developmental variant that has been reported to occur in 0.2–4% of the population [13–16]. However, coexistence of duplication of the inferior vena cava with the abdominal aortic aneurysm is described only in a few studies [5, 17–19], in which it accompanies other vascular variations [18] or developmental anomalies [20]. The duplicated inferior vena cava has a reported incidence of 2–3% in autopsy studies [15, 18]. However, this anomaly diagnosed by CT, was only 0.3–0.6% [13, 16]. This difference in occurrence suggests that the smaller component is not readily apparent on CT. Duplicated veins are typically thin-walled, dilated, and even may be tortuous [8, 17]. Such morphology may complicate surgical treatment and predispose the patient to unexpected bleeding. Embryological explanation of such developmental variation as duplication of the inferior vena cava is complex. During fetal development three segments constitute the inferior vena cava: the upper hepatic segment, the renal (subcardinal) segment, and the supracardinal (sacrocardinal) segment [21–23]. In 1925, McClure and Butler proposed the theory of inferior vena duplication [23]. It was modified by Larsen in 2001 [24]. According to their explanation

http://dx.doi.org/10.5772/66768

such an anomaly occurs due to failure of the caudal left supracardinal vein to regress resulting in an additional vein: the left inferior vena cava [23, 24].

Chen et al. [25] note that inferior vena cava anomalies were significantly more common in men than in women. A radiological study by Morita et al. [16] also found that such anomalies were significantly more common in men (39 of 3821 cases—1%) than in women (12 of 2473 cases—0.5%); men/women ratio is 2:1.

The knowledge of presence of a duplicated inferior vena cava in patient is clinically very important. It increases risk during abdominal aortic surgery [2]. The main reason is that anomalous veins are typically thin-walled, dilated, and therefore manipulation on them is challenging and at high risk of massive hemorrhage [6]. Probably, several small vessels at retroperotineal space may be injured during abdominal surgery. They are formed as rich collateral circulation compression of both the surrounding inferior vena cava by abdominal aortic aneurysm or atherosclerotic aorta [3]. Most commonly the left inferior vena cava ends as a junction with the left renal vein. They form a preaortic trunk, which opens to the right inferior vena cava [1, 10, 23, 25]. It existed in 67.9% of the cases with this variation [25]. In some examples, this junction is situated much lower and termed as the common iliac confluence [26, 27]. Sometimes the preaortic trunk was absent and the duplicated infrarenal left inferior vena ended as a left renal vein and with a reno-hemiazygos-lumbar trunk (RHLT) inserted into their junction [9, 28–30]. Knowledge on the duplication of the inferior vena cava with hemiazygos continuation of the left-sided IVC, preaortic trunk connection, and normal drainage of the right-sided IVC into the right atrium is also important from a hemodynamical point of view. Scrotal edema has already been described in patients with a duplication of the inferior vena cava, raising the question as to whether this anatomical variant is a predisposing factor [31].

Some studies speculate that duplication of the inferior vena cava may increase the incidence of thrombosis formation [7, 10–12]. Although the incidence of duplication of IVC is low, it certainly poses hazards during abdominal aortic aneurysm repair, and therefore endovascular treatment (EVAR) seems a safer choice than open surgery [9].

3. Retroaortic left renal vein

Usually, the human kidney is drained by several veins, which join near the hilum to form a single renal vein (RV). The left renal vein (LRV) passes anterior to the abdominal aorta and opens into the inferior vena cava (IVC) [32]. The morphology of the left renal vein (LRV) is much more complex than that of the right one because of its topography and relationship with the superior mesenteric artery and the abdominal aorta [33]. Also anomalies of the left renal vein are more common as those of the right renal vein because the left one is approximately three times longer and has a more complicated embryogenesis [34–36]. Knowledge about morphology of the left renal vein is especially important in transplantology because left kidney is preferred before donor nephrectomy [14, 37, 38].

One of the most common anomalies of the left renal vein is a retroaortic left renal vein (RLRV; **Figure 2**). It is located between the aorta and the vertebral column and drains into the inferior vena cava [32, 34]. This congenital anomaly occurs in 0.5–5.9% of the population according to the literature [14, 34, 39–41]. The retroaortic left renal vein was two times more frequent in females than in males [14]. However, according to Arslan et al. [42] and Nam et al. [43], the male to female ratio is similar.

The fourth and eighth gestational weeks are the time for development of the left renal vein. It is formed by the sequential formation, anastomoses, and regression of three paired veins (posterior cardinal, subcardinal, and supracardinal veins) [13, 14, 44]. At this time, there is an anastomotic junction between supracardinal and subcardinal channels, which produced a collar of veins around the aorta. When the ventral portion of the circumaortic collar persists, the normal left renal vein is formed. If the dorsal parts of this collar are persisted, the left renal vein passing posterior to the aorta produced a retroaortic left renal vein [34, 45, 46].

The retroaortic left renal vein is usually asymptomatic. However, its presence is clinically important [43]. Sometimes it may be due to clinical symptoms such as hematuria, abdominal/flank or inguinal pain, and vascular dilatations (varicocele) [34, 43, 47]. According to Karaman et al. [34], studying the frequency of the RLRV was significantly higher in the group with urological symptoms, especially in patients with hematuria, in comparison with the other group without urological symptoms. Heidler et al. [48] described that only 4 of 61 (6.6%) patient with RLRV diagnosed by CT scan were clinical symptomatic (flank pain and microhematuria).

The presence of a retroaortic left renal vein during the renal surgery influences the technical feasibility of the operation. Failure to recognize these anomalies may lead to non-suspected hemorrhage and even renal damage [43, 49]. Therefore, special attention in retroperitoneal space surgery is needed when retroaortic left renal vein is recognized. It seems especially important during an abdominal aortic aneurysm repair. Aortic dissection may be complicated by massive intraoperative bleeding, the most troublesome being venous rather than arterial hemorrhage [3]. Control of this bleeding is very difficult [3, 50]. Brener et al. [50] reported that during abdominal aortic reconstruction, approximately 40% of retroaortic left renal veins were injured. Of these, five were successfully repaired, two needed nephrectomy for control of the hemorrhage, and two patients died as a result of hemorrhage. Also the lumbar and retroperitoneal veins coalesce to form a complex retroaortic venous system whose topography and size depend on aortic aneurysm formation change and may be during dissection than the retroaortic LRV itself [3].

The fistula of the aorto-left renal vein in abdominal aortic aneurysms often co-occurs with the retroaortic left renal vein [51]. Mansour et al. [52] reported that 94% of the patients with aorto-left renal vein fistula also had a retroaortic left renal vein. Such complication is accompanied by hematuria, abdominal pain, left-sided varicocele, and a dysfunction of the left kidney [52–55]. A fistula probably forms due to the combination of the inflammatory process of the expanding abdominal aortic aneurysm and compression of the retroaortic left renal vein between the vertebral bodies and the pulsating aneurysm [53, 54]. Also inflammatory abdominal aortic aneurysm in patients with retroaortic left renal vein independently increases the complication rate during aortic surgery [56, 57].

Familiarity with the morphology of the main venous anomalies (especially including retroaortic and collar left renal vein) is the first step toward avoiding unexpected vascular injury during abdominal aortic procedures [3]. It seems important because coexistence nonruptured abdominal aortic aneurysm, with the prevalence of the retroaortic left renal vein estimated from 0.75 to 1.4% [2, 58].

4. Left renal vein collar

The circumaortic left renal vein (CLRV) or collar left renal vein is defined as the situation when this vein has an additional component that runs dorsal to the aorta and opens into the inferior vena cava (**Figure 3**) [32, 59]. According to statistics, the incidences of CLRV ranged 0.6–17.0% in cadaver dissection [60, 61], and 0.4–9.3% in clinical studies [47, 62]. In 2008, Natsis et al. [32] described a classification of the different forms of the circumaortic left renal vein based on the findings of 319 patients who underwent a CT angiography scan of the abdomen. The classification distinguished three types: Type I has one left renal vein splitting into two branches, a preaortic and a retroaortic, both of which opened into the inferior vena cava; Type II has two independent left renal veins, one preaortic and another retroaortic, draining into the inferior vena cava; Type III has existing anastomoses between the preaortic and retroaortic vein, being multiple or not, or multiple preaortic or retroaortic renal veins without anastomoses [32].

During the development of the inferior vena cava, there are anastomotic communications between supracardinal and subcardinal channels. The ventral portion of this connection persists as the normal left renal vein. If both the ventral and dorsal portions persist, the circumaortic (collar) left renal vein is formed [45, 46].

The CLRV in most cases is clinically silent and is discovered accidentally usually during Doppler ultrasonography, computed tomography, or magnetic imagining resonance. However, such information of presence of this variation is useful before abdominal surgery especially renal transplantation, caval interruption procedures, nephrectomy, portocaval shunts, and aortic aneurysm connective surgery [39, 63].

Morphology of the circumaortic left renal vein is important in abdominal aortic aneurysms because the retroaortic component of the circumaortic renal collar is usually thinner than the preaortic one and it is always located more caudally [32, 63, 64]. The vein may be damaged when the posterior stitches of the anastomosis are inserted resulting in severe bleeding or the formation of a graft-left renal vein fistula [3]. Abdominal aneurysm surgery poses a particular problem, because the LRV is used as a landmark below which the aorta is clamped [65]. During a retroperitoneal surgery, a preaortic vein is always visualized, but surgeon may be unaware of an additional retroaortic component or a posterior primary tributary and may avulse it while mobilizing the kidney or clamping the aorta [39, 66]. Also the relationship of circumaortic left renal vein to the ureter in the retroperitoneal space may be confusing, especially when aortic aneurysm is present and its topography has been changed [67].

The coexistence of an abdominal aortic aneurysm with RLRV or CLRV may also increase the probability of nutcracker syndrome [68]. The posterior type of nutcracer syndrome results in the narrowing of the LRV in its retroaortic or circumaortic position: compression between the aorta an`d the vertebral column [69, 70]. Therefore, the presence of an abdominal aortic aneurysm may also increase its symptoms and make treatment more dangerous.

5. Left-sided inferior vena cava

By definition, left-sided inferior vena cava, also known as transposition of the inferior vena cava, occurs when only one inferior vena cava is seen below the diaphragm on the left side of the abdominal aorta [71, 72]. A left IVC is thought to be caused by the regression of the right supracardinal vein with persistence of the left supracardinal vein during embryological development of the venous system [73]. The incidence of left-side inferior vena cava is 0.2–0.5% [74, 75]. According to Nishibe et al. [76], failure to recognize this variation when situated near the neck of the abdominal aortic aneurysm may lead LIVC injury and dangerous for live bleeding. Also proximal control of the neck of the aneurysm through a midline transperitoneal approach can be difficult if an anomalous inferior vena cava passes on the left side of aorta and crosses them during traveling to the right side of the body [2, 71]. Therefore, preoperative x-ray studies would be of value in this case [71, 77].

It is also important to remember that as a result of the transposition, the left adrenal and gonadal veins may empty directly into the left-sided inferior vena cava, while the right adrenal and gonadal veins drain into the right renal vein [78, 79].

6. Conclusion

Familiarity with the morphology of variations of the both left renal vein and inferior vena cava is important for all surgeons, urologists, and oncologists to reduce the risk of unexpected injury to these vessels. Such information is especially important when abdominal aortic aneurysm is present due to changes in the topography of the retroperitoneal space. If it is possible, a preoperative x-ray examination should be always performed in patients undergoing repair of the abdominal aortic aneurysm. All additional information precisely describing number and topography of vessels in retroperitoneal space prevents unexpected bleeding during surgical treatment of abdominal aortic aneurysm. Details of anomalous venous anatomy should be taken into consideration when choosing endovascular (EVAR) over classical treatment as the best and safest procedure.

Author details

Michał Polguj[1*], Katarzyna Stefańczyk[2] and Ludomir Stefańczyk[2]

*Address all correspondence to: michal.polguj@umed.lodz.pl

1 Department of Angiology, Medical University of Łódź, Łódź, Poland

2 Department of Radiology, Medical University of Łódź, Łódź, Poland

http://dx.doi.org/10.5772/66768

References

[1] Natsis K, Apostolidis S, Noussios G, Papathanasiou E, Kyriazidou A, Vyzas V. Duplication of the inferior vena cava: anatomy, embryology and classification proposal. Anat Sci Int 2010, 85: 56–60.

[2] Bartle EJ, Pearce WH, Sun JH, Rutherford RB. Infrarenal venous anomalies and aortic surgery: avoiding vascular injury. J Vasc Surg 1987, 6(6): 590–593.

[3] Karkos CD, Bruce IA, Thomson GJ, Lambert ME. Retroaortic left renal vein and its implications in abdominal aortic surgery. Ann Vasc Surg 2001, 15(6): 703–708.

[4] Nonami Y, Yamazaki M, Sato K, Sakamoto H, Ogoshi S. Two types of major venous anomalies associated with abdominal aneurysmectomy: a report of two cases. Surg Today 1996, 26(11): 940–944.

[5] Stefańczyk L, Majos M, Majos A, Polguj M. Duplication of the inferior vena cava and retroaortic left renal vein in a patient with large abdominal aortic aneurysm. Vasc Med 2014, 19(2): 144–145.

[6] Downey RS, Sicard GA, Anderson CB. Major retroperitoneal venous anomalies: surgical considerations. Surgery 1990, 107: 359–365.

[7] Nirupama A, Pallapothu R, Holmes R, Johnson MD. Inferior vena cava duplication and deep venous thrombosis: case report and review of literature. Ann Vasc Surg 2005, 19: 740–743.

[8] Polguj M, Majos M, Topol M, Majos A, Stefańczyk L. The influence of atherosclerotic abdominal aorta on the shape of duplicated inferior vena cava—its potential clinical implications and vascular complication. Folia Morphol 2014, 73(4): 521–526.

[9] Polguj M, Szubert W, Topol M, Stefańczyk L. An unusual duplication of the inferior vena cava in a patient with endovascular repair for abdominal aortic aneurysm. Rom J Morphol Embryol 2015, 56: 875–878.

[10] Bass JE, Redwine MD, Kramer LA, Huynh PT, Harris JH Jr. Spectrum of congenital anomalies of the inferior vena cava: cross-sectional imaging findings. Radiographics 2000, 20(3): 639–652.

[11] Cheng D, Zangan SM. Duplication of the inferior vena cava in a patient presenting for IVC filter placement. J Vasc Access 2010, 11(2): 162–164.

[12] Leong S, Oisin F, Barry JE, Maher MM, Bogue CO. Bilateral inferior vena cava filter insertion in a patient with duplication of the infrarenal vena cava. Ir J Med Sci 2012, 181(3): 389–391.

[13] Mayo J, Gray R, St Louis E, Grosman H, McLoughlin M, Wise D. Anomalies of the inferior vena cava. AJR Am J Roentgenol 1983, 140(2): 339–345.

[14] Dilli A, Ayaz UY, Kaplanoglu H, Saltas H, Hekimoglu B. Evaluation of the left renal vein variations and inferior vena cava variations by means of helical computed tomography. Clin Imaging 2013, 37: 530–535.

[15] Baldridge ED Jr, Canos AJ. Venous anomalies encountered in aortoiliac surgery. Arch Surg 1987, 122(10): 1184–1188.

[16] Morita S, Higuchi M, Saito N, Mitsuhashi N. Pelvic venous variations in patients with congenital inferior vena cava anomalies: classification with computed tomography. Acta Radiol 2007, 48(9): 974–979.

[17] Marrocco-Trischitta MM, Scicchitano G, Acconcia A, Stillo F. Management of synchronous abdominal aortic aneurysm and renal carcinoma associated with duplication of the inferior vena cava. J Cardiovasc Surg (Torino) 2001, 42(5): 683–685.

[18] Khaledpour C, Matanovic P, Rienäcker J, Grönniger J. An abdominal aortic aneurysm (AAA) in combination with duplication of the inferior vena cava (IVC), the right renal artery (RRA) and the right renal vein (RRV). Surg Radiol Anat 1990, 12(1): 73–76.

[19] Lee F, Quick CR. Abdominal aortic aneurysm associated with horseshoe kidney and duplication of inferior vena cava—an extra-peritoneal approach. Eur J Vasc Endovasc Surg 1997, 14(5): 406–407.

[20] Shaw MBK, Cutress M, Papavassiliou V, White S, Thompson M, Sayers R. Duplicated inferior vena cava and crossed renal ectopia with abdominal aortic aneurysm: preoperative anatomic studies facilitate surgery. Clin Anat 2003, 16(4): 355–357.

[21] Kellman GM, Alpern MB, Sandler MA, Craig BM. Computed tomography of vena caval anomalies with embryologic correlation. Radiographics 1988, 8(3): 533–556.

[22] Mathews R, Smith PA, Fishman EK, Marshall FF. Anomalies of the inferior vena cava and renal veins: embryologic and surgical considerations. Urology 1999, 53(5): 873–880.

[23] McClure CFW, Butler EG. The development of the vena cava inferior in man. Am J Anat 1925, 35(3): 331–383.

[24] Larsen WJ. Human embryology. 3rd edition, Churchill Livingstone, Philadelphia, 2001.

[25] Chen H, Emura S, Nagasaki S, Kubo KY. Double inferior vena cava with interiliac vein: a case report and literature review. Okajimas Folia Anat Jpn 2012, 88(4): 147–151.

[26] Colborn GL. A case of bilateral inferior vena cavae joined only at the iliac anastomosis. J Urol 1964, 91: 478–481.

[27] Pineda D, Moudgill N, Eisenberg J, DiMuzio P, Rao A. An interesting anatomic variant of inferior vena cava duplication: case report and review of the literature. Vascular 2013, 21(3): 163–167.

[28] Frantz P, Aboulker P, Küss R, Jardin A. Renal-rachidian venous trunk. Replacement of the left renal vein. A danger for the spinal cord. J Urol Nephrol (Paris) 1977, 83: 753–761.

[29] Scholbach T. From the nutcracker-phenomenon of the left renal vein to the midline congestion syndrome as a cause of migraine, headache, back and abdominal pain and functional disorders of pelvic organs. Med Hypotheses 2007, 68(6): 1318–1327.

[30] Brochert A, Reynolds T. Unusual duplication anomaly of the inferior vena cava with normal drainage of the right IVC and hemiazygous continuation of the left IVC. J Vasc Interv Radiol 2001, 12(12): 1453–1455.

[31] Itoh M, Moriyama H, Tokunaga Y, Miyamoto K, Nagata W, Satriotomo I, Shimada K, Takeuchi Y. Embryological consideration of drainage of the left testicular vein into the ipsilateral renal vein: analysis of cases of a double inferior vena cava. Int J Androl 2001, 24(3): 142–152.

[32] Natsis K, Tsitouridis I, Totlis T, Levva S, Tsikaras P, Skandalakis P. Proposal for classification of the circumaortic renal collar's morphology. Am Surg 2008 74(12): 1190–1194.

[33] Yi SQ, Ueno Y, Naito M, Ozaki N, Itoh M. The three most common variations of the left renal vein: a review and meta-analysis. Surg Radiol Anat 2012, 34(9): 799–804.

[34] Karaman B, Koplay M, Ozturk E, Basekim CC, Ogul H, Mutlu H, Kizilkaya E, Kantarci M. Retroaortic left renal vein: multidetector computed tomography angiography findings and its clinical importance. Acta Radiol 2007, 48(3): 355–360.

[35] Chuang VP, Mena CE, Hoskins PA. Congenital anomalies of the left renal vein: angiographic consideration. Br J Radiol 1974, 47: 214–218.

[36] Kraus GJ, Goerzer HG. MR-angiographic diagnosis of an aberrant retroaortic left renal vein and review of the literature. Clin Imaging 2003, 27: 132–134.

[37] Yagci B, Tavasli B, Karabulut N, Kiroglu Y. Clinical significance and renal haemodynamics of incidentally detected retroaortic left renal vein: assessment with venous Doppler sonography. Br J Radiol 2008, 81(963): 187–191.

[38] Turner RJ, Young SW, Castellino RA. Dynamic continuous computed tomography: study of retroaortic left renal vein. J Comput Assist Tomogr 1980, 4(1): 109–111.

[39] Satyapal KS, Kalideen JM, Haffejee AA, Singh B, Robbs JV. Left renal vein variations. Surg Radiol Anat 1999, 21(1): 77–81.

[40] Yesildag A, Adanir E, Köroglu M, Baykal B, Oyar O, Gülsoy UK. Incidence of left renal vein anomalies in routine abdominal CT scans. Tani Girisim Radyol 2004, 10(2): 140–143.

[41] Koc Z, Ulusan S, Oguzkurt L. Association of left renal vein variations and pelvic varices in abdominal MDCT. Eur Radiol 2007, 17: 1267–1274.

[42] Arslan H, Etlik O, Ceylan K, Temizoz O, Harman M, Kavan M. Incidence of retro-aortic left renal vein and its relationship with varicocele. Eur Radiol 2005, 15: 1717–1720.

[43] Nam JK, Park SW, Lee SD, Chung MK. The clinical significance of a retroaortic left renal vein. Korean J Urol 2010, 51(4): 276–280.

[44] Tore HG, Tatar I, Celik HH, Oto A, Aldur MM, Denk CC. Two cases of inferior vena cava duplication with their CT findings and a review of the literature. Folia Morphol 2005, 64(1): 55–58.

[45] Minniti S, Visentini S, Procacci C. Congenital anomalies of the venae cavae: embryological origin, imaging features and report of three new variants. Eur Radiol 2002, 12: 2040–2055.

[46] Turgut HB, Bircan MK, Hatipoglu ES, Dogruyol S. Congenital anomalies of left renal vein and its clinical importance: a case report and review of literature. Clin Anat 1996, 9: 133–135.

[47] Karazincir S, Balci A, Görür S, Sumbas H, Kiper AN. Incidence of the retroaortic left renal vein in patients with varicocele. J Ultrasound Med 2007, 26(5): 601–604.

[48] Heidler S, Hruby S, Schwarz S, Sellner-Zwieauer Y, Hoeltl W, Albrecht W. Prevelence and incidence of clinical symptoms of the retroaortic left renal vein. Urol Int 2015, 94: 173–176.

[49] Thomas TV. Surgical implications of retroaortic left renal vein. Arch Surg 1970, 100: 738–740.

[50] Brener BJ, Darling RC, Frederick PL, Linton RR. Major venous anomalies complicating abdominal aortic surgery. Arch Surg 1974, 108: 159–165.

[51] Tanaka H, Naito K, Murayama J, Ohteki H. Aorto-left renal vein fistula caused by a ruptured abdominal aortic aneurysm. Ann Vasc Dis 2013, 6(4): 738–740.

[52] Mansour MA, Rutherford RB, Metcalf RK, et al. Spontaneous aorto-left renal vein fistula: the "abdominal pain, hematuria, silent left kidney" syndrome. Surgery 1991, 109: 101–106.

[53] Yagdi T, Atay Y, Engin C, Ozbek SS, Buket S. Aorta-left renal vein fistula in a woman. Tex Heart Inst J 2004, 31: 435–438.

[54] Balduyck B, Van Den Brande F, Rutsaert R. Abdominal aortic aneurysm rupture into a retro-aortic left renal vein. Acta Chir Belg 2014, 114(2): 136–138.

[55] Barrier P, Otal P, Garcia O, Vahdat O, Domenech B, Lannareix V, Joffre F, Rousseau H. Aorta-left renal vein fistula complicating an aortic aneurysm: preoperative and postoperative multislice CT findings. Cardiovasc Intervent Radiol 2007, 30: 485–487.

[56] Bajardi G, Vitale G, Mirabella D, Bracale UM. Retroaortic left renal vein and inflammatory abdominal aortic aneurysm. Gen Thorac Cardiovasc Surg 2010, 58(4): 190–193.

[57] Lindblad B, Almgren B, Bergqvist B, Eriksson I, Forsberg O, Glimaker H, Jivegård L, Karlström L, Lundqvist B, Olofsson P. Abdominal aortic aneurysm with perianeurysmal fibrosis: experience from 11 Swedish vascular centers. J Vasc Surg 1991, 13: 231–237.

[58] Johnston KW, Scobie TK. Multicenter prospective study of nonruptured abdominal aortic aneurysms. I. Population and operative management. J Vasc Surg 1988, 7: 69–81.

[59] Beckmann CF, Abrams HL. Circumaortic venous ring: incidence and significance. AJR Am J Roentgenol 1979, 132: 561–565.

[60] Hoeltl W, Hruby W, Aharinejad S. Renal vein anatomy and its implications for retroperitoneal surgery. J Urol 1990, 143: 1108–1114.

[61] Anson BJ, Cauldwell EW. The pararenal vascular system a study of 425 anatomical specimens. Q Bull Northwest Univ Med Sch 1947, 21: 320–328.

[62] Costa HC, Moreira RJ, Fukunaga P, Fernandes RC, Boni RC, Matos AC. Anatomic variations in vascular and collecting systems of kidneys from deceased donors. Transplant Proc 2011, 43: 61–63.

[63] Satyapal KS. The renal veins: a review. Eur J Anatomy 2003, 7 (Suppl. 1): 43–52.

[64] Kramer B, Grine FE. The incidence of the renal venous collar in South African blacks. S Afr Med J 1980, 57: 875–876.

[65] Mitty HA. Circumaortic renal collar. A potentially hazardous anomaly of the left renal vein. Am J Roentgenol Radium Ther NucI Med 1975, 125: 307–310.

[66] Panagar AD, Subhash RL, Suresh BS, Nagaraj DN. Circumaortic left renal vein—a rare case report. J Clin Diagn Res. 2014, 8(3): 111–112.

[67] Kim MK, Ku YM, Chun CW, Lee SL. MDCT findings of right circumaortic renal vein with ectopic kidney. Korean J Radiol 2013, 14(5): 786–788.

[68] Wijdicks CA, Roseman DA. The clinical consequences of a circumaortic renal vein. Clin Anat 2007, 20(8): 986–987.

[69] Orczyk K, Łabętowicz P, Lodziński Sz, Stefańczyk L, Topol M, Polguj M. The nutcracker syndrome—morphology and clinical aspects of the important vascular variations: a systematic study of 112 cases. Intern Angiol 2016, 35(1): 71–77.

[70] Gulleroglu K, Gulleroglu B, Baskin E. Nutcracker syndrome. World J Nephrol 2014, 3: 277–281.

[71] Tsukamoto S, Shindo S, Obana M, Negishi N, Sezai Y. Operative management of abdominal aortic aneurysm with left-sided inferior vena cava. J Cardiovasc Surg (Torino) 2000, 41(2): 287–290.

[72] Davachi AA, Thomas J, Dale WA, Perry FA, Michael OB. Acute spontaneous rupture of an arteriosclerotic aneurysm into an isolated left-sided inferior vena cava. Am J Cardiol 1965, 15: 416–418.

[73] Allen C, Sauerland E, Sievert C, Bardin J. J Vasc Surg Venous Lymphat Disord 2014, 2(2): 206.

[74] Sarma KP. Anomalous inferior vena cava—Anatomical and clinical. Br J Surg 1966, 53: 600–602.

[75] Aljabri B, MacDonald PS, Satin R, Stein LS, Obrand DI, Steinmetz OK. Incidence of major venous and renal anomalies relevant to aortoiliac surgery as demonstrated by computed tomography. Ann Vasc Surg 2001, 15(6): 615–618.

[76] Nishibe T, Sato M, Kondo Y, Kaneko K, Muto A, Hoshino R, Kobayashi Y, Yamashita M, Ando M. Abdominal aortic aneurysm with left-sided inferior vena cava. Report of a case. Int Angiol 2004, 23(4): 400–402.

[77] Rispoli P, Conforti M, Cassatella R, Varetto G, Melloni CD, Raso AM. Left-sided inferior vena cava in patients submitted to aorto iliac surgery. Our experience and review of the literature. J Cardiovasc Surg (Torino) 2001 42(2): 249–255.

[78] Giordano JM, Trout HH. Anomalies of the inferior vena cava. J Vasc Surg 1986, 3: 924–928.

[79] Perler BA. Abdominal aortic replacement with a left-sided inferior vena cava: transperitoneal and left retroperitoneal approaches. J Cardiovasc Surg (Torino) 1989, 30(2): 236–240.

Chapter 9

Infected Aortic Aneurysms

Ting-Wei Lin and Chung-Dann Kan

Additional information is available at the end of the chapter

http://dx.doi.org/10.5772/66417

Abstract

Infected aortic aneurysms are surgical urgencies, requiring prompt management to avoid the development of catastrophic complications. Although traditional open surgery composed of radical debridement and aortic reconstruction remains the gold-standard, many favorable results of the endovascular repair strategy have been reported. In this chapter, the etiology, bacteriology, clinical manifestation, and diagnostic criteria of infected aortic aneurysms will be discussed in detail at first, followed by a comprehensive review of both traditional open surgery and endovascular repair, based on current evidences and the authors' institutional experience. Along with long-term oral antibiotic suppression and aggressive adjunctive procedures, endovascular repair for uncomplicated infected aortic aneurysms could be a definite treatment alternative to traditional open surgery in the endovascular era.

Keywords: infected aortic aneurysm, mycotic aortic aneurysm, antibiotic, aortic reconstruction, graft, endovascular aortic repair (EVAR), thoracic endovascular aortic repair (TEVAR)

1. Introduction

An infected aneurysm, commonly known as "mycotic aneurysm", is an abnormal dilatation of the artery associated with an infectious process [1–5]. In 1885, Sir William Osler first used the term "mycotic aneurysm" to describe multiple bead-like aneurysms of the aortic arch, resulting from suppuration in vessel wall in one patient with infective endocarditis-related aortic valve vegetations [1]. Currently, mycotic aneurysm is widely accepted as synonymous with infected aneurysm, describing all kinds of infected aneurysms with different etiologies, but not only those caused by septic emboli from a cardiac origin [6]. Moreover, the majority of infected (mycotic) aneurysms is caused by bacteria, but not fungus [4]. In this chapter, we will discuss in detail and review the current literatures about infected aneurysm, and we will present the authors' institutional experience of infected aneurysms involving the aorta. Here, the term "infected aortic aneurysm" instead of "mycotic aortic aneurysm" is used to prevent any misunderstanding.

Infected aortic aneurysms are generally surgical urgencies and comprise about 0.7–2.6% of all cases of aortic aneurysms [7–12]. The therapeutic considerations for infected aortic aneurysms include perioperative medical management (i.e., preoperative and postoperative antibiotic selection and course), timing and type of surgical procedures (traditional excision, debridement, and reconstruction versus endovascular technique), and the necessity of adjunctive procedures [7–15]. Complications occasionally occur at the initial presentation, including massive exsanguination due to free rupture and the development of aneurysm-related fistulations. Emergency operation is indispensable to salvage patients presenting with ruptured infected aortic aneurysms. Since the infectious process is usually not suppressed sufficiently even with proper antibiotic treatment course at the time of operation in these patients, the risk of postoperative persistent or even outbreak of infection is high [16–18]. Furthermore, the management of infected aortic aneurysms with aerodigestive communications is much more complex and remains inconclusive according to current evidence [18–23]. Thus, we will focus on uncomplicated infected aortic aneurysm in this chapter and propose strategies in managing this rare but severe disease in the endovascular era.

2. Etiology

Vascular infections with infected aneurysm formation generally have four types of etiologies according to Wilson's classification [4, 6]: (1) aneurysm formation after microbial arteritis due to bacteremia or local infection invasion, (2) posttraumatic infected pseudoaneurysms, which were usually related to drug abuse in the past and with increased incidence with the use of endovascular procedures [24] (3) infection of preexisting aneurysms, and (4) infected (mycotic) aneurysm resulting from infective endocarditis-related septic emboli (as described by Sir Osler) [1]. The intima of the arterial structure is normally resistant to infection; however, the presence of injury or pathological change makes it vulnerable to microorganisms, especially *Staphylococcus* and *Salmonella* species [25, 26]. Untreated local infection or arteritis that is not suppressed by host immunity in the early stage could progress to abscess formation, vascular perforation, and pseudoaneurysm formation. Furthermore, since the aorta is the most common site of atherosclerosis and aneurysm formation, infected aortic aneurysms usually result from bacteremic seeding to the diseased intima [6]. Rarely, infected aortic aneurysms secondary to an infectious process of adjacent structures, such as intraabdominal infection, empyema, mediastinitis, and vertebral osteomyelitis, have also been reported in Refs. [27–30].

Infected aortic aneurysms are also often developed in patients with various degrees of immunosuppressed status, such as in diabetes mellitus, liver cirrhosis, end-stage renal disease, alcoholism, chronic glucocorticoid therapy, chemotherapy, posttransplantation immunosuppression, human immunodeficiency virus infection, and malignancy [10, 31–34]. These patients frequently present with atypical clinical features that make the diagnosis difficult and uncommonly delayed [10]. In our institutional experience, more than 70% of the operated patients with infected aortic aneurysm had impaired immunity due to the aforementioned conditions at the time of operation.

3. Bacteriology

Overall, blood cultures were positive in more than half of patients with an infected aortic aneurysm, and intraoperative cultures could provide an even higher positive rate [5, 6, 35]. The causative microbiology of infected aortic aneurysms has changed after the advent of the antibiotic era and has a significant geographical difference. Before the popularized use of antibiotics, nonhemolytic *Streptococcus* species have once been the most common infectious organisms; subsequently, they account for less than 10% of infection cases after the advent of the antibiotic era [5, 36]. Currently, in Western countries, *Staphylococcus* species are generally the most common pathogens, accounting for 28–71% of cases based on published literatures [13, 37, 38]. It is also noteworthy that methicillin-resistant *Staphylococcus aureus* (MRSA) prevalence is continuously rising, and some reports indicated MRSA as the most dominant pathogen [39, 40]. Vancomycin-intermediate *Staphylococcus aureus* (VISA) has also been associated with infected aneurysms [41]. Gram-negative bacterium–related infected aortic aneurysms are less prevalent in Western countries than in East Asia, where *Salmonella* species are the most frequent Gram-negative bacteria causing aortic infections [11, 13, 38]. A diseased aorta, such as that with significant atherosclerotic change or preexisting aneurysm, is more vulnerable to *Salmonella* species [11]. In the literatures from Taiwan and in our institutional experience, *Salmonella* species account for 50–83% of cases of infected aortic aneurysms [11, 12, 14, 15].

Furthermore, the bacteriological spectrum may also be broader than that expected [37]. A recent report on endovascular treatment of infected aortic aneurysms from a European multicenter study revealed that 62% of the cases had a positive blood culture in which 20% was *Staphylococcus* species, 12% *Salmonella* species, and 11% *Streptococcus* species; approximately 19% were caused by other microorganisms [42]. A less common organism should always be considered in patients with infected aortic aneurysms, especially those in an immunosuppressed state [43]. Several Gram-negative bacterium–related infected aortic aneurysms have been described, including *Pseudomonas, Klebsiella, Escherichia coli, Campylobacter, Yersinia, Brucella, Haemophilus influenzae, Coxiella burnetii, Acinetobacter, Burkholderia pseudomallei, Campylobacter, Enterobacter cloacae,* and *Bacteroides fragilis* [44–55]. A Gram-negative bacterium–related infection is usually associated with more aneurysm rupture and mortalities. Moreover, infected aortic aneurysms due to various fungal infections have also been reported, such as *Candida, Cryptococcus,* and *Aspergillus* [56–58]. *Mycobacterium* species could also result in infected aortic aneurysms [59, 60], while *Bacillus* Calmette-Guérin–related abdominal aorta infection has also been reported in Ref. [61].

4. Clinical manifestation and diagnostic criteria

Unlike superficial infected aneurysms, which normally presents with painful, pulsatile masses along with local or systemic infection features, the clinical manifestation of infected aortic aneurysms is often obscure. Patients with an infected thoracic aortic aneurysm may have deep and vague chest or upper back pain, while those with infected abdominal aortic aneurysm may have abdominal or lower back pain. Oftentimes, patients with infected aortic aneurysms may only present with fever of unknown origin, and a diagnosis is made typically only after the aneurysms rupture or other complications develop. The structures adjacent to the infected aorta could be affected by direct bacterial invasion or a mass effect, resulting in gastrointestinal bleeding, dysphagia, hoarseness, hemoptysis, or the development of empyema, arteriovenous fistula, osteomyelitis, or psoas abscess [10, 62, 63].

The diagnosis of an infected aortic aneurysm is made by imaging studies and evidence of infection. Computed tomography (CT) angiography, which has been the diagnostic modality employed, could timely and clearly provide information on the size and location of the aneurysm as well as the anatomic relationship and possible involvement of the surrounding structures. The typical CT image suggestive of the presence of infectious process in the aorta shows irregular aortic wall, periaortic fat stranding, and presence of periaortic soft tissue mass, and fluid or air accumulation [64–66]. The aneurysm is usually saccular or multilobulated [65, 66]. Active extravasation of intravascular contrast medium is seen in ruptured aneurysm. A retropleural or retroperitoneal hematoma formation adjacent to the aneurysm can be observed if the aneurysm has a contained rupture. If contrast medium exposure is contraindicated, magnetic resonance angiography is the alternative choice of imaging study. As previously mentioned, it is not uncommon that no microorganism is identified in the blood sample from patients with infected aortic aneurysms; thus, a negative blood culture could not exclude the presence of infected aortic aneurysms.

Moreover, an infected aortic aneurysm should be distinguished from an inflammatory aortic aneurysm, although not always easy especially considering that both have the following clinical symptoms: chest, abdominal, or back pain and low-grade fever. The presence of positive serial antinuclear antibody (ANA) and elevated IgG4 in patients with aortitis or aortic aneurysm could imply an underlying autoimmune disease [67, 68]. A "mantle sign" on CT imaging is suspicious of an inflammatory aortic aneurysm, which displays a thickened wall of the aortic aneurysm with periaortic inflammation and fibrosis [67].

5. Management

Infected aneurysms are clinically serious, and those involving the aorta could result in more significant morbidity and mortality despite prompt surgical interventions. With the high percentage of disease evolution to aneurysm rupture, antibiotic treatment alone results in extremely poor prognoses and should be only reserved for those with very high surgical risk and significant medical comorbidities [69]. Aggressive debridement with aortic reconstruction remains the gold-standard operative procedure; however, a complicated postoperative course generally could be anticipated [7]. Furthermore, for infected aneurysms affecting the thoracic aorta and aortic arch, the surgical procedure typically employs extracorporeal circulation, cardiopulmonary bypass, and even a period of deep hypothermic circulatory arrest (DHCA), further increasing the operative risks. The feasibility of endovascular aortic repair (EVAR) for infected aortic aneurysms has been investigated in numerous studies, which in turn provided encouraging short-term results [18, 42, 70–74]. However, the long-term survival and late-onset complications, especially recurrent or persistent infections, are of greater concerns [74].

5.1. Antibiotic therapy

If an infected aortic aneurysm is suspected clinically, systemic broad-spectrum antibiotics should be initiated immediately before definite pathogen identification [69, 75]. Because of the high prevalence of *Salmonella* species infection in our country, we prefer administering ceftriaxone in every case of an infected aortic aneurysm if there is no contraindication [12, 69, 71]. Once the culture and susceptibility results are available, antibiotics should be tailored accordingly. The minimum inhibitory concentration (MIC) of every susceptible antibiotic should be assessed and specialist consultation for infectious diseases should be liberal.

The optimal duration of antibiotic therapy both before and after surgical repair of an infected aortic aneurysm remains inconclusive. Generally, 4–8 weeks of systemic antibiotic course is accepted as the minimum treatment duration for infected aortic aneurysms [75]. The treatment effectiveness should be assessed, and the therapeutic course should be based on subsequent blood culture, serial examination of the inflammatory markers, and persistent evaluation of the clinical progress. Patients infected with highly drug-resistant organisms usually require a longer antibiotic therapy duration [76]. Furthermore, since the infected aorta is generally either reconstructed by prosthetic graft implantation or repaired with endovascular prosthesis deployment, suppressive oral antibiotics for a prolonged period following completed parenteral antibiotic therapy is often warranted [18, 69, 77]. Further details of the antibiotic therapy will be discussed in Sections 7.2 and 7.5.

5.2. Traditional open repair

Open surgical repair for an infected aortic aneurysm is composed of excision of the diseased aorta, debridement of the surrounding infected tissue, and immediate, and usually in situ, reconstruction of the aortic continuity. This operation technique for infected aortic aneurysms is generally consistent with that for noninfected aortic aneurysms. Patient positioning and surgical exposure depend on the anatomical and pathological conditions of the aneurysm, and the adjunctive monitoring or protective measures should be prudently executed based on the consensus between the surgeon and anesthesiologist. The operative considerations for infected aortic aneurysms with different anatomical locations are discussed below, and some representative completed reconstructions are illustrated in **Figure 1**.

5.2.1. Infected ascending aortic and aortic arch aneurysms

To replace an infected aneurysm of the ascending aorta and aortic arch, cardiopulmonary bypass is absolutely required, and an interval of DHCA is often necessary. Electroencephalographic monitoring or continuous recording of cerebral oxygen saturation is advisable. Intraoperative transesophageal echocardiography (TEE) is performed to assess cardiac function [78]. A full median sternotomy is the standard approach, and an extension to the neck or even a "trap-door" incision is sometimes needed for better exposure of the distal arch and its branches. If aortic valve replacement is necessary for infective endocarditis or a concomitant pathology of the aortic valve, a composite graft replacement, or a separated replacement of the valve and aorta, is performed. Coronary arteries are reimplanted to the prosthetic graft with buttons of the aorta tissue (Button-Bentall procedure) if the aortic root is replaced [79, 80]. Occasionally,

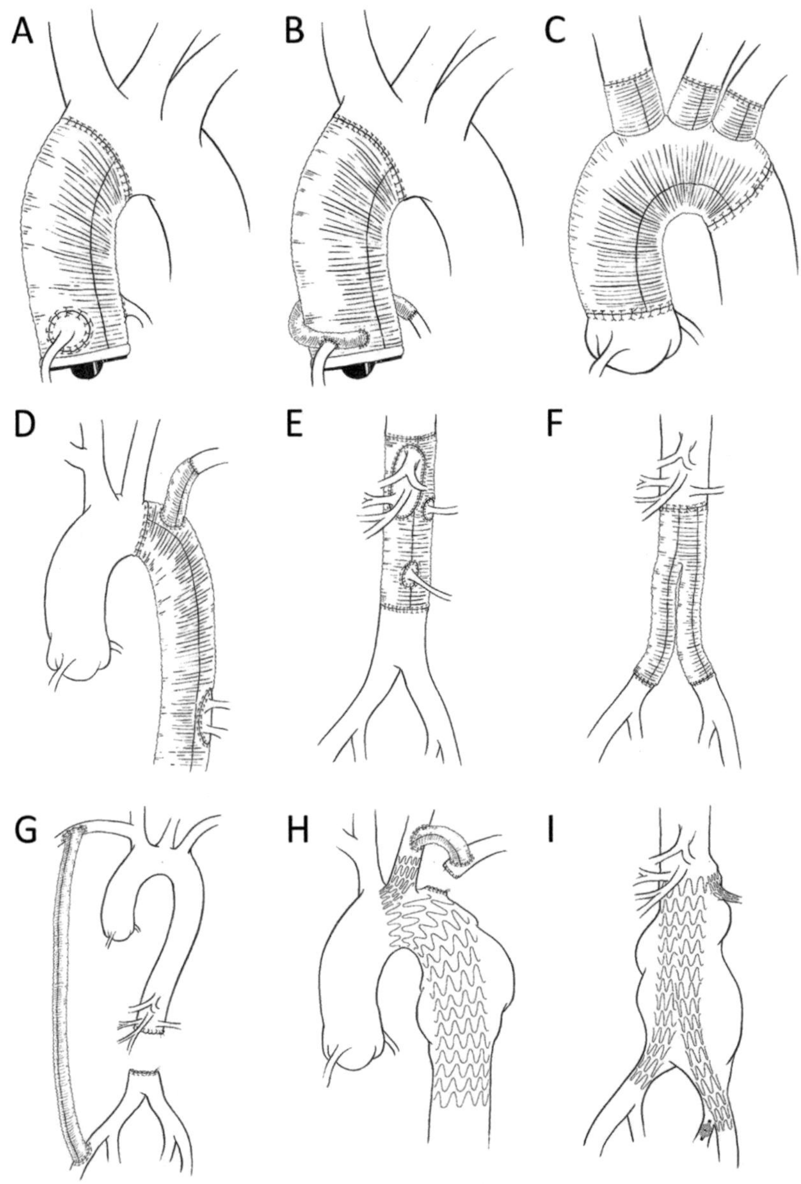

Figure 1. Illustrations of different aortic reconstructions. (A) Ascending aorta and aortic root replacement, with a composite graft with a mechanical valve and reimplantation of the coronary arteries with buttons of the aorta tissue (Button-Bentall procedure). (B) Ascending aorta and aortic root replacement, with a composite graft with Cabrol modification. (C) Total arch replacement. (D) Descending thoracic aorta and proximal left subclavian artery replacement (semi-arch replacement), with reimplantation of the important spinal arteries (e.g., Adamkiewicz artery). (E) Juxta-renal abdominal aorta replacement, with reimplantation of all visceral arteries. (F) Infra-renal abdominal aorta and iliac arteries replacement, with a bifurcated graft. Note the inferior mesenteric artery is not reimplanted. (G) Axillo-femoral bypass (extra-anatomical reconstruction), with aortic stumps closure. (H) Thoracic endovascular aortic repair (TEVAR), with chimney technique for left carotid artery debranching and a carotid-subclavian bypass for proximal sealing zone at zone I. (I) Endovascular aortic repair (EVAR), with chimney technique for left renal artery debranching and plug embolization for left internal iliac artery.

http://dx.doi.org/10.5772/66417

no adequate healthy tissue for coronary artery reimplantation is found; a Cabrol technique or coronary artery bypass graft (CABG) can be used to reestablish the coronary flow [81, 82].

5.2.2. *Infected thoracic and thoracoabdominal aortic aneurysms*

Similar to noninfected thoracic and thoracoabdominal aortic aneurysms, an infected thoracic aortic aneurysm is repaired through a left thoracotomy with suitable intercostal spaces or a more extended thoracoabdominal incision [11, 77]. A simple clamp-and-sew technique, partial cardiopulmonary bypass, or left heart bypass can be chosen according to the characteristics of the aneurysm and the preference of the surgical team. If there is no space for proximal clamping, proximal anastomosis under a period of DHCA is necessary, and the use of intraoperative cerebral monitoring is also advisable. Cerebrospinal fluid (CSF) drainage should be routinely performed in all suitable patients, and evoked potential measurement should be considered [83, 84]. If the operation is performed with simple aortic clamping, some adjunctive protective measures in addition to CSF drainage could be done, such as hypothermia (cool the patient to 34°C or slightly lower with low operation room temperature or cold intravenous fluid) and cold renal perfusion with crystalloid or blood [77, 83–85]. Of note, the adoption of clamp-and-sew technique during an infected thoracic aortic aneurysm repair should be carefully evaluated because excising the infected aorta and performing debridement often takes a considerably more time, which increases the distal ischemic time despite the utilization of various protective strategies.

5.2.3. *Infected abdominal (juxta-renal, supra-renal, and infra-renal) aortic aneurysms*

Infected abdominal aortic aneurysms are generally repaired using a simple clamp-and-sew method through a median laparotomy, without extracorporeal circulatory support [9, 86]. Renal protective measures as previously described should be considered for those with a juxta-renal or supra-renal location. The involved visceral arteries are reimplanted to the graft [87]. Historically, aortic reconstruction with an autologous femoropopliteal venous graft has been advocated [88]. The time consumed and the morbidities caused by femoropopliteal vein harvest, along with the lack of availability of cryopreserved allografts, have urged more surgeons to prefer using prosthetic grafts, usually a Dacron graft, as alternatives [12, 14, 89–91]. An omental flap with preserved vascular supply is usually transposed to cover the graft and the anastomosis sites. Omental flaps separate the prosthesis from the surrounding contaminated structures and fill a dead space. The highly vascularized flap could also facilitate the systemic antibiotic delivery to the infected area [14].

5.2.4. *Extra-anatomical reconstruction*

To avoid prosthetic graft placement in the contaminated field and to restore the aortic flow with a remote route, extra-anatomical reconstruction is an attractive alternative to in situ reconstruction [9, 87, 92, 93]. Extra-anatomical reconstruction also includes excision of the infected aorta and debridement of the surrounding contaminated tissue, with aortic stump closure and aortic revascularization through a noninfected pathway. A unilateral or bilateral axillo-femoral bypass after an infra-renal abdominal aorta excision is the most common procedure. Extra-anatomical reconstruction has also been used for the repair of infected aneurysm of the aortic arch [94]. Because of the residual aortic tissue fragility, a sustained risk of aortic stump disruption exists [87, 95]. A two-layer closure is generally recommended, with coverage of a vascularized omental flap.

5.3. Endovascular technique

Since the first report by Semba et al. [96], an increasing number of investigations on endovascular technique utilization in infected aortic aneurysm management, including one European multicenter study published in 2014 [15, 18, 42, 70–74, 97, 98], was noted. The general principle and considerations of endovascular treatment for infected aortic aneurysms are identical to those for noninfected aortic aneurysms, including consideration of the characteristics of each device, arterial access route assessment (usually the iliac and femoral artery), anatomical characteristics of the aneurysm, and proximal and distal sealing zones.

A high-resolution multi-slice CT angiography providing essential information and a well-reconstructed three-dimensional image is usually necessary for surgical planning. The endovascular procedure is performed in a hybrid operating room equipped with a fluoroscopic unit, where prompt conversion to traditional open surgery is possible. Depending on the patient's situation, the procedure could be performed under general anesthesia, spinal anesthesia, or even local anesthesia. For patients with long-segment descending thoracic aorta coverage by the stent graft or, ideally for all patients undergoing thoracic endovascular aortic repair (TEVAR), CSF drainage should be performed for neuroprotection [99, 100]. Although controversial, the artery of Adamkiewicz, normally located between T8 and L2, should be preserved if possible [100]. If essential branches of the aorta are to be covered by stent grafts, revascularization by either a bypass surgery, open debranching, or endovascular debranching with a chimney technique or a fenestrated stent graft is necessary [101–105]. Adjunctive procedures, such as open debridement and percutaneous drainage, could be performed, based on the clinical judgment [74].

Although endovascular treatment for ascending aortic pathologies, including those with an infectious process, has been sporadically investigated [106–109], its use remains "off-label" for current commercially available aortic stent grafts. Further advances in the design of the devices and well-constructed studies are both necessary. Consequently, endovascular management for infected ascending aortic aneurysms is not discussed herein.

6. Outcomes

6.1. Antibiotic therapy alone

It was believed that patients with infected aortic aneurysms treated medically without undergoing aortic resection surviving to hospital discharge is almost impossible [38, 69]. In 2009, Hsu and colleagues from Taiwan reported the institutional experience of medical treatment of infected aortic aneurysms in high-risk patients, which revealed that the prognosis was not uniformly fatal [69]. The treatment strategy is composed of 6–8 weeks parenteral antibiotic administration during hospitalization, followed by lifelong oral antibiotics. Of the 22 patients (8 thoracic and 14 abdominal aortic aneurysms), the overall in-hospital mortality rate was 50% and the 1-year event-free survival rate was 32%. Ruptured aneurysm was the major cause of death, accounting for 40.9% (9/22) of patients treated medically. Of note, two in-hospital deaths due to massive gastrointestinal tract bleeding, whose etiology was not mentioned, were reported; aortoesophageal or aortoenteric fistulations could be the possible causes. The most common causative agent was the *Salmonella* species, which is responsible for 50% (11/22) of the cases, and the authors found that the prognosis of medically treated *Salmonella*-infected aneurysms was better than that of non-*Salmonella* infected cases. However, the prognosis of medically treated *Salmonella*-infected aortic aneurysm remains a subject of debate as most of the early reports from Western countries showed an extremely dismal result [38, 110, 111] (see more details in Section 7.1). The authors concluded that although the results of antibiotic treatment alone in patients with infected aortic aneurysm remained poor, it could still be an alternative treatment, especially in *Salmonella*-infected patients with very high surgical risks.

6.2. Traditional open repair

Due to the rarity of the disease, most reports regarding the surgical outcome of infected aortic aneurysms after traditional open repair have very heterogeneous case characteristics, with various aortic segments involved and different methods for aortic reconstruction [9–14, 16, 17, 77, 112–118]. Although admirable surgical outcomes have been reported, with both early and late mortalities as low as 5%, an early mortality rate of 5–40% and an at least 30% late mortality rate after open surgical repair of infected aortic aneurysms were demonstrated in most literatures [9–14, 16, 17, 77, 112–118]. Generally, the surgical outcomes for infected aneurysms with an infrarenal location were better than those involving the aortic arch and descending thoracic, thoracoabdominal, supra-renal, and juxta-renal aorta [11, 13, 16, 116]. An infected aneurysm of the ascending aorta is rare, and a successful surgical treatment has been reported in Refs. [119–123].

More than 50% of the patients undergoing open surgical repair of infected aortic aneurysms had early major complications, such as acute kidney injury, respiratory failure, and spinal ischemia. Late vascular complications, mostly a prosthetic graft infection, developed in up to 30% of the survivors [9–14, 16, 17, 77, 112–118]. Although the late outcomes are similar between in situ and extra-anatomical reconstruction, the latter is related to higher vascular complications, including aortic stump disruption (8–19%) and limb amputation (17–27%) [91–95]. Re-infection of the prosthetic graft is also possible in patients undergoing extra-anatomical reconstruction [93, 95]. Nevertheless, extra-anatomical reconstruction is still a reasonable option for patients who are unsuitable for in situ reconstruction.

6.3. Endovascular technique

The short-term advantage of endovascular infected aortic aneurysm repair has been gradually clarified, although most reports comprise small case numbers and limited follow-ups [15, 70–74, 97, 98]. In 2007, Kan and colleagues reviewed English literatures investigating the efficiency of EVAR for infected aortic aneurysms [18]. The estimated overall 30-day survival rate was 89.6%, and the 2-year survival rate was 82.2% for the extracted 48 cases. Ruptured aneurysm, including those complicated with aortic fistulations, and fever at the time of EVAR procedure were found to be the significant predictors of persistent infection. Several studies continuously demonstrated that EVAR is a possible alternative procedure for infected aortic aneurysm patients with high surgical risks, with an early mortality rate less than 20%, which is comparable to that of traditional open repair. A poorer outcome was still evident in patients with aneurysm-related fistulation complication [71, 72, 124–127]. Persistent infection greatly contributed to both early and late mortalities; thus, adjunctive procedures to eliminate contamination and prolonged antibiotic therapy duration after EVAR were usually advocated in the literatures [18, 72, 74] (see more details in Sections 7.4 and 7.5).

In 2014, Sörelius and colleagues conducted a European multicenter study, the largest retrospective study, to investigate the durability of EVAR for infected aortic aneurysms [42]. The 30-day, 1-year, 5-year, and 10-year survival rate of the 123 patients identified was 91, 75, 55, and 41%, respectively. Of note, infected aortic aneurysms caused by non-*Salmonella* microorganisms were identified to have a worse long-term prognosis. Location of the aneurysm, presence of shock, or ruptured aneurysm at the time of operation showed no effects on the late outcome. Aneurysm-related infection complications developed in 33 patients (26.83%) postoperatively, 23 of whom had an either early or late lethal outcome. The authors concluded that EVAR could be a feasible and durable choice for most patients with infected aortic aneurysms. Persistent or recurrent infection remained a great concern, necessitating a long-term antibiotic therapy and regular follow-up.

6.3.1. The institutional experience of endovascular management for uncomplicated infected aortic aneurysms from National Cheng Kung University Hospital, Tainan, Taiwan

National Cheng Kung University Hospital is a tertiary medical center in southern Taiwan and serves as a first-line hospital in Tainan City with an urban population of 1.8 million and also as a referral center for the whole southern Taiwan. As of the writing of this manuscript, a total of 338 EVAR procedures (including TEVAR and hybrid procedures) for various purposes have been performed.

Since the first case of infected thoracic aortic aneurysm treated by TEVAR in March 2009, 25 patients have undergone endovascular management for infected aortic aneurysms in our hospital. Six complicated cases were excluded from this study: two presented with aneurysm-free rupture and hemorrhagic shock and received emergency EVAR and four were associated with aortoesophageal or aortobronchial fistulas. Finally, 19 cases, with a mean age of 68.68 years (range: 43.94–83.65 years) and a mean follow-up of 20.54 months (range: 0.59–85.13 months), were included. Several valuable preoperative and postoperative images from selected patients are shown in (**Figures 2–5**). There was one in-hospital mortality that had persistent periaortic graft infection despite continuous parenteral antibiotic treatment.

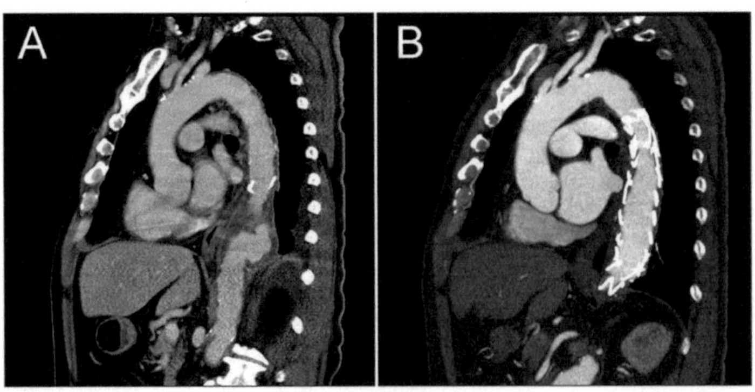

Figure 2. (A) Infected descending thoracic aortic aneurysm in a 70-year-old male patient (B) Oral antibiotic treatment continued for 1 year after TEVAR and CT angiography 2 years after TEVAR showed no residual aneurysm or periaortic infection. No adjunctive procedure was ever done for this patient.

http://dx.doi.org/10.5772/66417

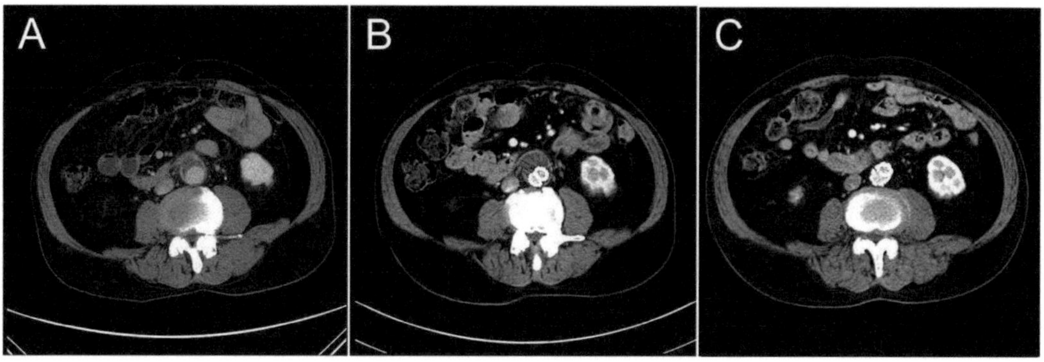

Figure 3. (A) Infected infra-renal abdominal aortic aneurysm in a 68-year-old diabetic male patient (B) CT angiography 2 weeks after EVAR showed residual aneurysm but resolved periaortic inflammation. Percutaneous drainage of the aneurysm was done. (C) With long-term oral antibiotic suppression, the aneurysm disappeared completely on CT angiography 2 years later.

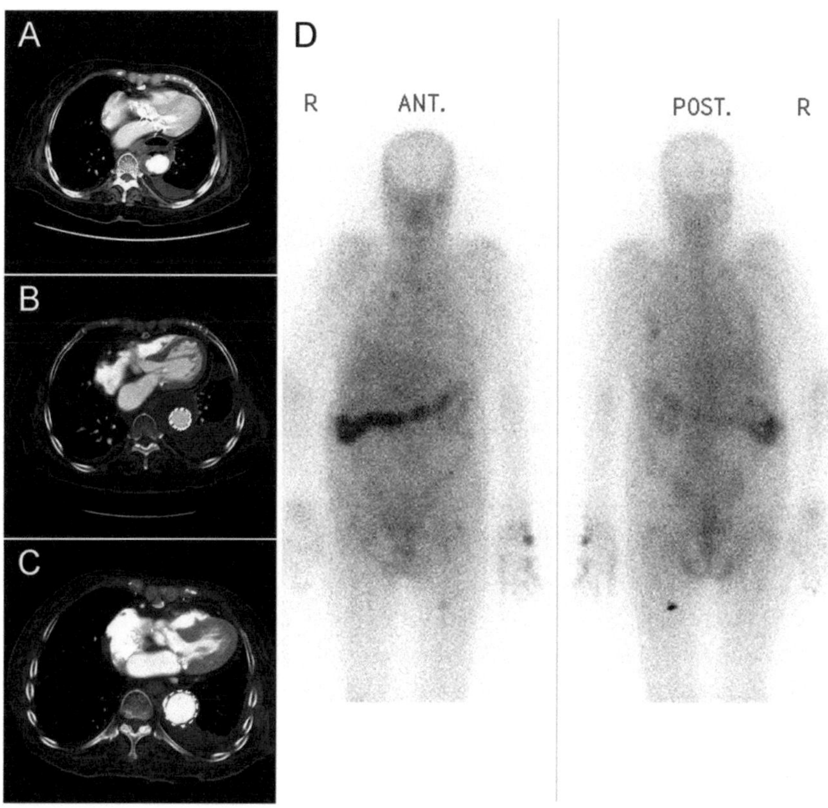

Figure 4. (A) Infected descending thoracic aortic aneurysm with periaortic foamy air collection (emphysematous aortitis) in an 83-year-old diabetic female patient. (B) Two weeks after TEVAR, there was still fluid accumulation around the stent graft and also abundant pleural effusion. Debridement through left mini-thoracotomy was done. (C) With long-term oral antibiotic suppression, the periaortic inflammation resolved 6 months later, despite this there was still some pleural effusion. (D) Gallium inflammation scan confirmed that there was no residual infection process.

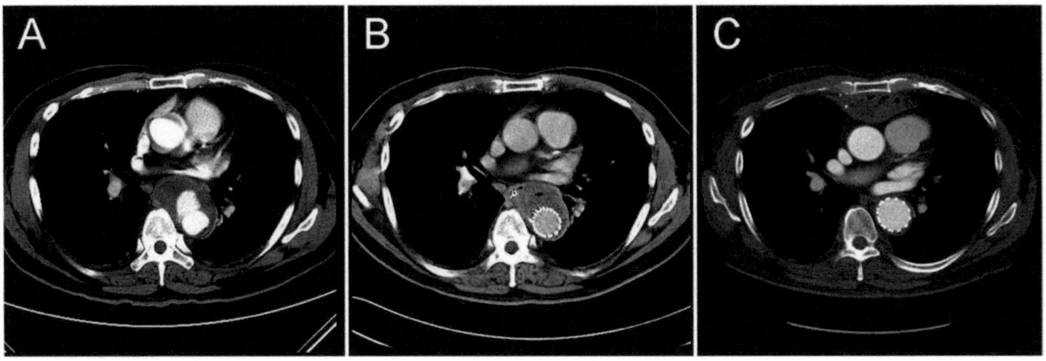

Figure 5. (A) Infected descending thoracic aortic aneurysm caused by *Salmonella enteritidis* in a 60-year-old male patient. (B) The patient was complicated with persistent local infection and esophageal perforation 1 week after TEVAR. Debridement and esophagectomy by a video-assisted thoracic surgery (VATS) was done. (C) Oral antibiotics were kept for 1 year after hospital discharge and CT angiography 3 years after TEVAR showed completely resolved periaortic infection. Note the retrosternal gastric tube for esophagus reconstruction.

The patient refused open debridement and died 2 months after the EVAR procedure. Major postoperative early complications developed in nine patients (47.37%), including respiratory failure requiring tracheostomy in four, acute kidney injury in three, esophageal perforation in two, spinal cord ischemia in one, lower extremity ischemia in one, and hypoxic encephalopathy in one. The two cases developing esophageal perforation had no hematemesis at initial presentation and their preoperative CT angiographies did not reveal any feature of aortoesophageal fistula. Persistent local infection or ischemic esophageal necrosis after TEVAR should be the cause resulting in esophageal perforation. Both these patients underwent subsequent radical debridement and esophagectomy and were alive during the last follow-up.

Three late mortalities occurred, of which one was aneurysm-related mortality. The patient developed recurrent periaortic infection and subsequent aortoenteric fistula 2 years after the operation and died because of massive exsanguination. The estimated 30-day, 1-year, and 5-year aneurysm-related survival rate was 100, 94.1, and 78.4%, respectively. No endoleak was detected by CT angiography beyond 30 days postoperatively. All patients with a follow-up duration more than 6 months had disappearance of aneurysms along with complete resolution of periaortic inflammation.

Long-term antibiotics were prescribed in nine patients (47.37%) in the study population. Adjunctive procedures to eliminate the infectious environment were performed in seven patients (36.84%), including open debridement in four (two patients also underwent concomitant esophagectomy for postoperative esophageal perforation as previously mentioned) and percutaneous drainage in three patients. Due to the rarity of both early and late mortalities, the evaluation of the benefit of long antibiotic therapy duration and adjunctive procedures is challenging. For the same reason, analysis of other predictors of inferior early and late outcomes was not performed.

7. Controversies

7.1. *Salmonella*-related versus non-*Salmonella*-related infected aortic aneurysm

Infected aortic aneurysms caused by *Salmonella* species were thought to be more virulent and tend to have a worse outcome, in view of the higher risk of early aneurysm rupture and prosthetic graft infection [110, 111, 128–132]. In 2010, Kan and colleagues compared the surgical outcomes of 41 cases of infected aortic aneurysms identified from relevant literature reports and institute cases from 1990 to 2008 and found that *Salmonella* infection was a risk factor of postoperative aneurysm-related morbidity and mortality [71]; however, the type of procedures (i.e., traditional open repair versus EVAR) was not.

With the advent of effective modern antibiotics, improved outcomes of *Salmonella*-related infected aortic aneurysms were reported in most of the recent literatures [12, 15, 118]. *Salmonella* infection prevalence in our institution is high; thus, we routinely prescribe ceftriaxone as one of the empiric antibiotic agents (usually, vancomycin or oxacillin is added for a better coverage of Gram-positive microorganisms), provided that no contraindications are noted, once a diagnosis of an infected aortic aneurysm was made even before the availability of definite culture result. We also found a favorable outcome in patients with infected aortic aneurysms caused by *Salmonella* species in our institution. On the other hand, some studies identified a positive culture of non-*Salmonella* species as a predictor of a poorer outcome after both open surgery and endovascular procedures [17, 42, 77]. Thus, although still inconclusive, *Salmonella* infection should at least not be considered as a predictor of a worse outcome for infected aortic aneurysm.

7.2. Preoperative antibiotic course

Infected aortic aneurysms are surgical urgencies, and our mentors used to inculcate in us the cliché "avoid undue delay of operation." Nevertheless, implanting a vascular prosthesis into a contaminated field in a patient with an active systemic infection might result in a catastrophic graft infection. Thus, the usual practice is to perform the operation after a period of parenteral antibiotic treatment if the patient's condition permits [17, 18, 77, 116].

Hsu and colleagues retrospectively analyzed the clinical outcome of infected aortic aneurysms in National Taiwan University Hospital, Taipei, Taiwan, from 1995 to 2011 [118]. Of the 109 patients identified, 85 underwent surgical intervention, including open repair in 77 and endovascular repair in eight. The median preoperative antibiotic treatment duration was 8 days (interquartile range: 2–21 days). Ten deaths (early or late) directly related to persistent/recurrent periaortic infection or prosthesis infection were reported. The authors found that shorter preoperative antibiotic treatment duration was associated with more aneurysm-related moralities: a median preoperative antibiotic duration of 3 days (interquartile range: 0–7 days) in the deceased and 16 days (interquartile range: 3–26 days) in the survivors. In the systemic review of infected aortic aneurysms treated with EVAR by Kan et al. [18], 22 of the 48 patients received preoperative antibiotics for more than 1 week, and two patients had a postoperative persistent infection. In the univariate analysis, preoperative antibiotic treatment more than 1 week had a protective effect against persistent infection; however, its benefit was not significant in the multivariate analysis. In fact, the decision on the preoperative antibiotic course is highly determined by other clinical conditions, which in turn could be confounding factors for worse prognosis. For example, the presence of aneurysm-related complications or profound sepsis would urge the surgeon to perform operation earlier, and both situations could affect the surgical outcome.

No study investigating the optimal surgical timing for infected aortic aneurysms after initial antibiotic treatment has so far been conducted; thus, the ideal preoperative antibiotic treatment duration remains controversial. If the clinical condition permits, we favor performing operation (either open or endovascular repair) at least when fever subsides after adequate systemic parenteral antibiotic treatment or, more desirably, after a 7-day antibiotic course or confirmation of a negative culture result.

7.3. Choice of graft materials for in situ reconstruction

Numerous graft materials to reestablish the aortic continuity in situ are available, such as a prosthetic graft, an autologous venous graft, a cryopreserved allograft, and even an autologous or xenologous pericardial patch [91, 117, 133, 134]. An autologous venous graft or an allograft was considered to be more resistant to microorganisms than a prosthetic graft and thus used to be the preferred material for infected aorta reconstruction [88]. Despite the low reinfection rate and good durability of the autologous femoropopliteal venous grafts, considerable major morbidities are associated with femoropopliteal vein harvest, including compartment syndrome requiring fasciotomy in 12% and chronic venous insufficiency in 15% of the patients [89]. The availability of cryopreserved allografts in Taiwan and most countries in East Asia is limited [14, 117].

The reinfection rate after in situ reconstruction with prosthetic grafts for infected aortic aneurysms, which was as high as 20% in early reports [135], has decreased significantly recently. Several studies in Taiwan, including our institutional experience, have demonstrated a graft infection rate of 8.0–10.4% after in situ prosthetic graft replacement for infected aortic aneurysms [11, 12, 113–116, 118]. In a more recent study investigating the outcomes of open repair of infected descending thoracic and thoracoabdominal aortic aneurysms by Lau et al., no postoperative graft infection occurred in 14 patients who had in situ prosthetic graft reconstruction [77].

In 2011, Bisdas et al. analyzed the prognosis of cryopreserved allografts and silver-coated Dacron grafts for abdominal aortic infections with positive intraoperative culture and found comparable short-term and mid-term survival rates [91]. None of the 22 patients in the cryopreserved allograft group developed graft infection, while two of the 11 patients in the silver-coated Dacron graft group had an ongoing or recurrent infection. Of interest, the costs of therapy were significantly higher for cryopreserved allografts. Moreover, other studies have revealed favorable results of in situ antibiotic-bonded prosthetic graft replacement for infected aortic aneurysms [117, 136]; nevertheless, its effectiveness still requires further investigations.

7.4. Adjunctive procedures after the initial EVAR

The major concern of endovascular treatment for infected aortic aneurysms is the residual infectious environment surrounding the deployed device. Additional surgical procedures, such as debridement of the infected tissue and drainage of the abscess, could aid in eradicating the infection and thus improve the outcome [18, 74, 137]. Furthermore, additional culture information could be obtained through the specimen derived from these procedures.

In our systemic review, performing adjunctive procedures after EVAR serves as a protective factor against persistent infection in the univariate analysis; however, the benefit was insignificant in the multivariate analysis [18]. In 2011, Kritpracha and colleagues published their institutional experience of endovascular therapy for infected aortic aneurysms and showed an impressive mid-term outcome for those without an aortic fistulation [72]. They routinely prescribed lifelong antibiotics to the patients, and no adjunctive procedure was conducted. During a mean follow-up of 22 months, no late mortality or aneurysm-related complication in the 15 patients surviving to hospital discharge was reported. Complete resolution of periaortic inflammation and shrinkage of the aneurysms were observed in most of the patients starting at the 6-month follow-up. The authors thus suggested that aggressive debridement of the infected tissue may not be necessary for those with uncomplicated infected aortic aneurysms.

Determining the effectiveness of each adjunctive procedure is also difficult, and the selection should be individualized. We prefer performing CT-guided drainage if the patient remains febrile or unsterilized blood sample persists after EVAR provided that the periaortic abscess has been adequately liquefied. Irrigation of the abscess cavity with antibiotics or disinfectants could also be performed [74]. A more extensive open debridement is generally reserved for those with an unsatisfactory response to the aforementioned less-invasive measures.

7.5. Postoperative antibiotic course

No consensus on the optimal postoperative antibiotic treatment duration is available. For other cardiovascular infections, at least 4–8 weeks of parenteral antibiotic therapy after surgical intervention is generally accepted, and the course should be carefully tailored according to the clinical and laboratory parameters [75]. Several authors have advocated long-term oral antibiotic suppression after hospital discharge for all operated patients, especially those who underwent endovascular repair [9, 10, 15, 42, 77]. However, drug adherence is typically less than ideal, mainly because of the development of antibiotic-related adverse reactions or patient noncompliance.

In the early institutional experience of in situ prosthetic graft replacement for infected abdominal aortic aneurysms published in 2003, Luo and colleagues found that oral antibiotic suppression, prolonged or not, was not related to the development of late graft infection [12]. Thereafter, we did not routinely prescribe oral antibiotics to patients who had received open repair at hospital discharge. Following our strategy of both pre- and postoperative antibiotic treatment, as previously mentioned, only two patients have developed late graft infections after in situ prosthetic graft replacement for infected abdominal aortic aneurysms [14].

Moreover, in our practice, long-term oral antibiotic suppression is generally planned at hospital discharge for those who had endovascular repair for infected aortic aneurysms [15]. The surgeon's decision on antibiotic treatment termination, provided that no residual infection based on clinical, imaging, and laboratory evidence is noted, is individualized. Of 18 hospital survivors with uncomplicated infected aortic aneurysms treated with EVAR, along with long-term oral antibiotic suppression and aggressive adjunctive procedures, only one patient (5.6%) developed a late aneurysm-related complication (i.e., recurrent periaortic infection complicated with aortoenteric fistula).

8. Epilogue

Based on current evidence and our institutional experience, we have introduced and adopted the following therapeutic strategy for infected aortic aneurysms in the endovascular era:

1. Open repair through the excision of the infected aorta and radical debridement of the surrounding contaminated structure with immediate aortic reconstruction remains the gold standard. Although a higher reinfection rate is theoretically possible, in situ reconstruction with a prosthetic graft, along with adequate perioperative antibiotic course, is a safe and durable choice and could be applied in most patients. Long-term oral antibiotic suppression is not necessary provided that no evidence of ongoing infection after completion of parenteral antibiotic therapy is found.

2. For uncomplicated infected aortic aneurysms, endovascular treatment can be a reasonable alternative, especially for patients with significant comorbidities. If clinically feasible, an EVAR procedure can be performed after controlling overt infection, usually at least 3–7 days after parenteral broad-spectrum antibiotic treatment. The postoperative parenteral antibiotic treatment duration is at least 4–8 weeks. Long-term or even lifelong oral antibiotic suppression is recommended, and adjunctive procedures to eliminate the infectious environment are also considered. With the adoption of the abovementioned therapeutic strategies, the role of EVAR for uncomplicated infected aortic aneurysms has evolved from a temporary palliation to a reliable definite therapy.

Acknowledgements

This work is supported by funding from Medical Science and Technology Research Grant, National Cheng Kung University Hospital (NCKUH-10506021).

Author details

Ting-Wei Lin and Chung-Dann Kan*

* Address all correspondence to: kcd56@mail.ncku.edu.tw

Division of Cardiovascular Surgery, Department of Surgery, National Cheng Kung University Hospital, College of Medicine, Tainan, Taiwan

References

[1] Osler W. The Gulstonian lectures, on malignant endocarditis. Br Med J. 1885;1:467-470. DOI: 10.1136/bmj.1.1262.467.

[2] Revell S. Primary mycotic aneurysms. Ann Intern Med. 1945;22:431-440. DOI: 10.7326/0003-4819-22-3-431.

[3] Anderson CB, Butcher HR Jr, Ballinger WF. Mycotic aneurysms. Arch Surg. 1974;109:712-717. DOI: 10.1001/archsurg.1974.01360050106022.

[4] Wilson SE, Van Wagenen P, Passaro E Jr. Arterial infection. Curr Probl Surg. 1978;15:1-89. DOI: 10.1016/s0011-3840(78)80003-3.

[5] Johnson JR, Ledgerwood AM, Lucas CE. Mycotic aneurysm. New concepts in therapy. Arch Surg. 1983;118:577-582. DOI: 10.1001/archsurg.1983.01390050053010.

[6] Patel S, Johnston KW. Classification and management of mycotic aneurysms. Surg Gynecol Obstetr. 1977;144:691-694.

[7] Reddy DJ, Shepard AD, Evans JR, Wright DJ, Smith RF, Ernst CB. Management of infected aortoiliac aneurysms. Arch Surg. 1991;126:873-878. DOI: 10.1001/archsurg.1991.01410310083012.

[8] Beck AW, Velazquez-Ramirez G. Infected aneurysms. In: Cronenwett JL, Johnston KW, editors. Rutherford's vascular surgery. 8th ed., Philadelphia: Springer; 2014. pp.2236-2247.

[9] Müller BT, Wegener OR, Grabitz K, Pillny M, Thomas L, Sandmann W. Mycotic aneurysms of the thoracic and abdominal aorta and iliac arteries: experience with anatomic and extra-anatomic repair in 33 cases. J Vasc Surg. 2001;33:106-113. DOI: 10.1067/mva.2001.110356.

[10] Oderich GS, Panneton JM, Bower TC, Cherry KJ Jr, Rowland CM, Noel AA, Hallett JW Jr, Gloviczki P. Infected aortic aneurysms: aggressive presentation, complicated early outcome, but durable results. J Vasc Surg. 2001;34:900-908. DOI: 10.1067/mva.2001.118084.

[11] Hsu RB, Tsay YG, Wang SS, Chu SH. Surgical treatment for primary infected aneurysm of the descending thoracic aorta, abdominal aorta, and iliac arteries. J Vasc Surg. 2002;36:746-750. DOI: 10.1067/mva.2002.126557.

[12] Luo CY, Ko WC, Kan CD, Lin PY, Yang YJ. In situ reconstruction of septic aortic pseudoaneurysm due to Salmonella or Streptococcus microbial aortitis: long-term follow-up. J Vasc Surg. 2003;38:975-982. DOI: 10.1016/s0741-5214(03)00549-4.

[13] Moneta GL, Taylor LM Jr, Yeager RA, Edwards JM, Nicoloff AD, McConnell DB, Porter JM. Surgical treatment of infected aortic aneurysm. Am J Surg. 1998;175:396-399. DOI: 10.1016/s0002-9610(98)00056-7.

[14] Lai CH, Luo CY, Lin PY, Kan CD, Chang RS, Wu HL, Yang YJ. Surgical consideration of in situ prosthetic replacement for primary infected abdominal aortic aneurysms. Eur J Vasc Endovasc Surg. 2011;42:617-624. DOI: 10.1016/j.ejvs.2011.07.005.

[15] Kan CD, Yen HT, Kan CB, Yang YJ. The feasibility of endovascular aortic repair strategy in treating infected aortic aneurysms. J Vasc Surg. 2012;55:55-60. DOI: 10.1016/j.jvs.2011.07.077.

[16] Fillmore AJ, Valentine RJ. Surgical mortality in patients with infected aortic aneurysms. J Am Coll Surg. 2003;196:435-441. DOI: 10.1016/s1072-7515(02)01607-1.

[17] Hsu RB, Chen RJ, Wang SS, Chu SH. Infected aortic aneurysms: clinical outcome and risk factor analysis. J Vasc Surg. 2004;40:30-35. DOI: 10.1016/j.jvs.2004.03.020.

[18] Kan CD, Lee HL, Yang YJ. Outcome after endovascular stent graft treatment for mycotic aortic aneurysm: a systematic review. J Vasc Surg. 2007;46:906-912. DOI: 10.1016/j.jvs.2007.07.025.

[19] Canaud L, Ozdemir BA, Bee WW, Bahia S, Holt P, Thompson M. Thoracic endovascular aortic repair in management of aortoesophageal fistulas. J Vasc Surg. 2014;59:248-254. DOI: 10.1016/j.jvs.2013.07.117.

[20] Okita Y, Yamanaka K, Okada K, Matsumori M, Inoue T, Fukase K, Sakamoto T, Miyahara S, Shirasaka T, Izawa N, Ohara T, Nomura Y, Nakai H, Gotake Y, Kano H. Strategies for the treatment of aorto-oesophageal fistula. Eur J Cardiothorac Surg. 2014;46:894-900. DOI: 10.1093/ejcts/ezu094.

[21] Mosquera VX, Marini M, Pombo-Felipe F, Gómez-Martinez P, Velasco C, Herrera-Noreña JM, Cuenca-Castillo JJ. Predictors of outcome and different management of aortobronchial and aortoesophageal fistulas. J Thorac Cardiovasc Surg. 2014;148:3020-3026. DOI: 10.1016/j.jtcvs.2014.05.038.

[22] Canaud L, D'Annoville T, Ozdemir BA, Marty-Ané C, Alric P. Combined endovascular and surgical approach for aortobronchial fistula. J Thorac Cardiovasc Surg. 2014;148:2108-2111. DOI: 10.1016/j.jtcvs.2014.01.018.

[23] Czerny M, Reser D, Eggebrecht H, Janata K, Sodeck G, Etz C, Luehr M, Verzini F, Loschi D, Chiesa R, Melissano G, Kahlberg A, Amabile P, Harringer W, Janosi RA, Erbel R, Schmidli J, Tozzi P, Okita Y, Canaud L, Khoynezhad A, Maritati G, Cao P, Kölbel T, Trimarchi S. Aorto-bronchial and aorto-pulmonary fistulation after thoracic endovascular aortic repair: an analysis from the European Registry of Endovascular Aortic Repair Complications. Eur J Cardiothorac Surg. 2015;48:252-257. DOI: 10.1093/ejcts/ezu443.

[24] Pipkin W, Brophy C, Nesbit R, Mondy Iii JS. Early experience with infectious complications of percutaneous femoral artery closure devices. J Vasc Surg. 2000;32:205-208. DOI: 10.1067/mva.2000.105678.

[25] Sommerville Rl, Allen Ev, Edwards Je. Bland and infected arteriosclerotic abdominal aortic aneurysms: a clinicopathologic study. Medicine (Baltimore). 1959;38:207-221. DOI: 10.1097/00005792-195909000-00001.

[26] Sedivy P, Sebesta P, Trejbalová E, Henysová J. Infected false aneurysm caused by hematogenous dissemination of Staphylococcus aureus after the use of vaginal tampons. Int Angiol. 2008;27:439-441.

[27] Garb M. Appendicitis: an unusual cause of infected abdominal aortic aneurysm. Australas Radiol. 1994;38:68-69. DOI: 10.1111/j.1440-1673.1994.tb00132.x.

[28] Fraser CD 3rd, Arnaoutakis GJ, George TJ, Owens JB, Conte JV, Shah AS. Acute cholecystitis preceding mycotic aortic pseudoaneurysm in a heart transplant recipient. J Card Surg. 2010;25:749-51. DOI: 10.1111/j.1540-8191.2010.01138.x.

[29] Learch TJ, Sakamoto B, Ling AC, Donovan SM. Salmonella spondylodiscitis associated with a mycotic abdominal aortic aneurysm and paravertebral abscess. Emerg Radiol. 2009;16:147-150. DOI: 10.1007/s10140-008-0713-6.

[30] Chen SH, Lin WC, Lee CH, Chou WY. Spontaneous infective spondylitis and mycotic aneurysm: incidence, risk factors, outcome and management experience. Eur Spine J. 2008;17:439-444. DOI: 10.1007/s00586-007-0551-3.

[31] Kaneko K, Nonomura Y, Watanabe K, Koike R, Kubota T, Harigai M, Inoue Y, Iwai T, Miyasaka N. Infected abdominal aortic aneurysm caused by nontyphoid Salmonella in an immunocompromised patient with rheumatoid arthritis. J Infect Chemother. 2009;15:312-315. DOI: 10.1007/s10156-009-0699-3.

[32] Bowden DJ, Hayes PD, Sadat U, Choon See T. Mycotic pseudoaneurysm of the superficial femoral artery in a patient with Cushing disease: case report and literature review. Vascular. 2009;17:163-167. DOI: 10.2310/6670.2008.00060

[33] Sharma K, Kibria R, Ali S, Rao P. Primary aortoenteric fistula caused by an infected abdominal aortic aneurysm with Mycobacterium avium complex in an HIV patient. Acta Gastroenterol Belg. 2010;73:280-282.

[34] Gunst JD, Jensen-Fangel S. A mycotic abdominal aortic aneurysm caused by Listeria monocytogenes in a patient with HIV infection. BMJ Case Rep. 2014;2014. DOI: 10.1136/bcr-2013-202712.

[35] Maeda H, Umezawa H, Goshima M, Hattori T, Nakamura T, Umeda T, Shiono M. Primary infected abdominal aortic aneurysm: surgical procedures, early mortality rates, and a survey of the prevalence of infectious organisms over a 30-year period. Surg Today. 2011;41:346-351. DOI: 10.1007/s00595-010-4279-z.

[36] Cartery C, Astudillo L, Deelchand A, Moskovitch G, Sailler L, Bossavy JP, Arlet P. Abdominal infectious aortitis caused by Streptococcus pneumoniae: a case report and literature review. Ann Vasc Surg. 2011;25:266.e9-e16. DOI: 10.1016/j.avsg.2010.07.014.

[37] Brossier J, Lesprit P, Marzelle J, Allaire E, Becquemin JP, Desgranges P. New bacteriological patterns in primary infected aorto-iliac aneurysms: a single-centre experience. Eur J Vasc Endovasc Surg. 2010;40:582-588. DOI: 10.1016/j.ejvs.2010.07.020.

[38] Brown SL, Busuttil RW, Baker JD, Machleder HI, Moore WS, Barker WF. Bacteriologic and surgical determinants of survival in patients with mycotic aneurysms. J Vasc Surg. 1984;1:541-547. DOI: 10.1067/mva.1984.avs0010541.

[39] Utsumi T, Ohtsuka M, Uchida E, Yamaguchi H, Nakajima T, Akazawa H, Takano H, Nakaya H, Komuro I. Abdominal aortic pseudoaneurysm caused by prolonged methicillin-resistant Staphylococcus aureus sepsis. Int J Cardiol. 2008;128:294-295. DOI: 10.1016/j.ijcard.2007.06.043.

[40] Karkos CD, Burnett C, Buckely H, Sheen AJ, Williams GT. Mycotic common iliac artery aneurysm complicating methicillin-resistant Staphylococcus aureus bacteremia: an unusual cause of ureteric obstruction. Ann Vasc Surg. 2005;19:904-908. DOI: 10.1007/s10016-005-7686-7.

[41] Kuo CC, Wu V, Tsai CW, Chou NK, Wang SS, Hsueh PR. Fatal bacteremic mycotic aneurysm complicated by acute renal failure caused by daptomycin-nonsusceptible, vancomycin-intermediate, and methicillin-resistant Staphylococcus aureus. Clin Infect Dis. 2008;47:859-860. DOI: 10.1086/591280.

[42] Sörelius K, Mani K, Björck M, Sedivy P, Wahlgren CM, Taylor P, Clough RE, Lyons O, Thompson M, Brownrigg J, Ivancev K, Davis M, Jenkins MP, Jaffer U, Bown M, Rancic Z, Mayer D, Brunkwall J, Gawenda M, Kölbel T, Jean-Baptiste E, Moll F, Berger P, Liapis CD, Moulakakis KG, Langenskiöld M, Roos H, Larzon T, Pirouzram A, Wanhainen A, European MAA collaborators. Endovascular treatment of mycotic aortic aneurysms: a European multicenter study. Circulation. 2014;130:2136-2142. DOI: 10.1161/CIRCULATIONAHA.114.009481.

[43] Jarrett F, Darling RC, Mundth ED, Austen WG. Experience with infected aneurysms of the abdominal aorta. Arch Surg. 1975;110:1281-1286. DOI: 10.1001/archsurg.1975.01360170021002.

[44] Dick J, Tiwari A, Menon J, Hamilton G. Abdominal aortic aneurysm secondary to infection with Pseudomonas aeruginosa: a rare cause of mycotic aneurysm. Ann Vasc Surg. 2010;24:692. e1-e4. DOI: 10.1016/j.avsg.2010.02.003.

[45] Hsu RB, Lin FY. Psoas abscess in patients with an infected aortic aneurysm. J Vasc Surg. 2007;46:230-235. DOI: 10.1016/j.jvs.2007.04.017.

[46] McCann JF, Fareed A, Reddy S, Cheesbrough J, Woodford N, Lau S. Multi-resistant *Escherichia coli* and mycotic aneurysm: two case reports. J Med Case Rep. 2009;3:6453. DOI: 10.1186/1752-1947-3-6453.

[47] Hadou T, Elfarra M, Alauzet C, Guinet F, Lozniewski A, Lion C. Abdominal aortic aneurysm infected by Yersinia pseudotuberculosis. J Clin Microbiol. 2006;44:3457-3458. DOI: 10.1128/JCM.00486-06.

[48] Park SJ, Kim MN, Kwon TW. Infected abdominal aortic aneurysm caused by Brucella abortus: a case report. J Vasc Surg. 2007;46:1277-1279. DOI: 10.1016/j.jvs.2007.06.043.

[49] Takahashi Y, Tsutsumi Y, Monta O, Kohshi K, Ohashi H. Mycotic aneurysm of the descending thoracic aorta caused by *Haemophilus influenzae*. J Card Surg. 2010;25:218-220. DOI: 10.1111/j.1540-8191.2009.00990.x.

[50] Bendermacher BL, Peppelenbosch AG, Daemen JW, Oude Lashof AM, Jacobs MJ. Q fever (*Coxiella burnetii*) causing an infected thoracoabdominal aortic aneurysm. J Vasc Surg. 2011;53:1402-1404. DOI: 10.1016/j.jvs.2010.11.102.

[51] Lee SY, Sin YK, Kurup A, Agasthian T, Caleb MG. Stent-graft for recurrent melioidosis mycotic aortic aneurysm. Asian Cardiovasc Thorac Ann. 2006;14:e38-e40. DOI: 10.1177/021849230601400232.

[52] Rao J, Kaushal AS, Hoong CK. Abdominal aortic pseudoaneurysm secondary to melioidosis. Asian J Surg. 2009;32:64-69. DOI: 10.1016/S1015-9584(09)60012-9.

[53] Hagiya H, Matsumoto M, Furukawa H, Murase T, Otsuka F. Mycotic abdominal aortic aneurysm caused by Campylobacter fetus: a case report and literature review. Ann Vasc Surg. 2014;28:1933.e7-1933.e14. DOI: 10.1016/j.avsg.2014.06.072.

[54] Tanaka K, Kawauchi M, Murota Y, Furuse A. 'No-Touch' isolation procedure for ruptured mycotic abdominal aortic aneurysm. Jpn Circ J. 2001;65:1085-1086. DOI: 10.1253/jcj.65.1085.

[55] Lee HL, Liu KH, Yang YJ, Kan CD. *Bacteroides fragilis* aortic arch pseudoaneurysm: case report with review. J Cardiothorac Surg. 2008;3:29. DOI: 10.1186/1749-8090-3-29.

[56] Brunner S, Engelmann MG, Näbauer M. Thoracic mycotic pseudoaneurysm from *Candida albicans* infection. Eur Heart J. 2008;29:1515. DOI: 10.1093/eurheartj/ehm623.

[57] Deitch JS, Plonk GW, Hagenstad C, Hansen KJ, Peacock JE Jr, Ligush J Jr. Cryptococcal aortitis presenting as a ruptured mycotic abdominal aortic aneurysm. J Vasc Surg. 1999;30:189-192. DOI: 10.1016/s0741-5214(99)70191-6.

[58] Mettananda KC, De Silva ST, Premawardhena AP. Mycotic aneurysm of the descending aorta due to Aspergillus species. Ceylon Med J. 2010;55:20-21. DOI: 10.4038/cmj.v55i1.1705.

[59] Long R, Guzman R, Greenberg H, Safneck J, Hershfield E. Tuberculous mycotic aneurysm of the aorta: review of published medical and surgical experience. Chest. 1999;115:522-531. DOI: 10.1378/chest.115.2.522.

[60] Canaud L, Marzelle J, Bassinet L, Carrié AS, Desgranges P, Becquemin JP. Tuberculous aneurysms of the abdominal aorta. J Vasc Surg. 2008;48:1012-1016. DOI: 10.1016/j.jvs.2008.05.012.

[61] Harding GE, Lawlor DK. Ruptured mycotic abdominal aortic aneurysm secondary to Mycobacterium bovis after intravesical treatment with bacillus Calmette-Guérin. J Vasc Surg. 2007;46:131-134. DOI: 10.1016/j.jvs.2007.01.054.

[62] Skourtis G, Papacharalambous G, Makris S, Kasfikis F, Kastrisios G, Goulas S, Antoniou I, Giannakakis S, Maltezos C. Primary aortoenteric fistula due to septic aortitis. Ann Vasc Surg. 2010;24:825.e7-e11. DOI: 10.1016/j.avsg.2010.02.030.

[63] Yamamoto H, Yamamoto F, Izumoto H, Tanaka F, Ishibashi K. Repetitive contained rupture of an infected abdominal aortic aneurysm with concomitant vertebral erosion. Ann Vasc Surg. 2010;24:824.e1-e5. DOI: 10.1016/j.avsg.2010.02.024.

[64] Wu HY, Kan CD. Images in cardiovascular medicine: Emphysematous aortitis. Circulation. 2010;122:e413. DOI: 10.1161/CIRCULATIONAHA.109.924001.

[65] Lee WK, Mossop PJ, Little AF, Fitt GJ, Vrazas JI, Hoang JK, Hennessy OF. Infected (mycotic) aneurysms: spectrum of imaging appearances and management. Radiographics. 2008;28:1853-1868. DOI: 10.1148/rg.287085054.

[66] Lai CH, Chang RS, Luo CY, Kan CD, Lin PY, Yang YJ. Mycotic aneurysms in the abdominal aorta and iliac arteries: CT-based grading and correlation with surgical outcomes. World J Surg. 2013;37:671-679. DOI: 10.1007/s00268-012-1850-3.

[67] Pennell RC, Hollier LH, Lie JT, Bernatz PE, Joyce JW, Pairolero PC, Cherry KJ, Hallett JW. Inflammatory abdominal aortic aneurysms: a thirty-year review. J Vasc Surg 1985;2:859-869. DOI: 10.1067/mva.1985.avs0020859.

[68] Ishizaka N, Sohmiya K, Miyamura M, Umeda T, Tsuji M, Katsumata T, Miyata T. Infected aortic aneurysm and inflammatory aortic aneurysm – in search of an optimal differential diagnosis. J Cardiol. 2012;59:123-131. DOI: 10.1016/j.jjcc.2011.10.006.

[69] Hsu RB, Chang CI, Wu IH, Lin FY. Selective medical treatment of infected aneurysms of the aorta in high risk patients. J Vasc Surg. 2009;49:66-70. DOI: 10.1016/j.jvs.2008.08.004.

[70] Patel HJ, Williams DM, Upchurch GR Jr, Dasika NL, Eliason JL, Deeb GM. Late outcomes of endovascular aortic repair for the infected thoracic aorta. Ann Thorac Surg. 2009;87:1366-1371. DOI: 10.1016/j.athoracsur.2009.02.030.

[71] Kan CD, Lee HL, Luo CY, Yang YJ. The efficacy of aortic stent grafts in the management of mycotic abdominal aortic aneurysm-institute case management with systemic literature comparison. Ann Vasc Surg. 2010;24:433-440. DOI: 10.1016/j.avsg.2009.08.004.

[72] Kritpracha B, Premprabha D, Sungsiri J, Tantarattanapong W, Rookkapan S, Juntarapatin P. Endovascular therapy for infected aortic aneurysms. J Vasc Surg. 2011;54:1259-1265. DOI: 10.1016/j.jvs.2011.03.301.

[73] Sedivy P, Spacek M, El Samman K, Belohlavek O, Mach T, Jindrak V, Rohn V, Stadler P. Endovascular treatment of infected aortic aneurysms. Eur J Vasc Endovasc Surg. 2012;44:385-394. DOI: 10.1016/j.ejvs.2012.07.011.

[74] Tsai MT, Kan CD. Following the short-term benefit of endovascular repair of mycotic aortic aneurysm: what is the next step? J Endovasc Ther. 2013;20:311-314. DOI: 10.1583/13-4222C.1.

[75] Chan FY, Crawford ES, Coselli JS, Safi HJ, Williams TW Jr. In situ prosthetic graft replacement for mycotic aneurysm of the aorta. Ann Thorac Surg. 1989;47:193-203. DOI: 10.1016/0003-4975(89)90268-3.

[76] Cinà CS, Arena GO, Fiture AO, Clase CM, Doobay B. Ruptured mycotic thoracoabdominal aortic aneurysms: a report of three cases and a systematic review. J Vasc Surg. 2001;33:861-867. DOI: 10.1067/mva.2001.111977.

[77] Lau C, Gaudino M, de Biasi AR, Munjal M, Girardi LN. Outcomes of open repair of mycotic descending thoracic and thoracoabdominal aortic aneurysms. Ann Thorac Surg. 2015;100:1712-1717. DOI: 10.1016/j.athoracsur.2015.05.067.

[78] Bryan AJ, Barzilai B, Kouchoukos NT. Transesophageal echocardiography and adult cardiac operations. Ann Thorac Surg. 1995;59:773-779. DOI: 10.1016/0003-4975(94)00818-3.

[79] Bentall H, De Bono A. A technique for complete replacement of the ascending aorta. Thorax 1968;23:338-339. DOI: 10.1136/thx.23.4.338.

[80] Lewis CT, Cooley DA, Murphy MC, Talledo O, Vega D. Surgical repair of aortic root aneurysms in 280 patients. Ann Thorac Surg. 1992;53:38-45. DOI: 10.1016/0003-4975(92)90755-S.

[81] Cabrol C, Pavie A, Gandjbakhch I, Villemot JP, Guiraudon G, Laughlin L, Etievent P, Cham B. Complete replacement of the ascending aorta with reimplantation of the coronary arteries: new surgical approach. J Thorac Cardiovasc Surg. 1981;81:309-315.

[82] Rokkas CK, Kouchoukos NT. Surgical management of the severely atherosclerotic ascending aorta during cardiac operations. Semin Thorac Cardiovasc Surg. 1998;10:240-246. DOI: 10.1016/s1043-0679(98)70024-3.

[83] Safi HJ, Hess KR, Randel M, Iliopoulos DC, Baldwin JC, Mootha RK, Shenaq SS, Sheinbaum R, Greene T. Cerebrospinal fluid drainage and distal aortic perfusion: reducing neurologic complications in repair of thoracoabdominal aortic aneurysm types I and II. J Vasc Surg. 1996;23:223-229. DOI: 10.1016/s0741-5214(96)70266-5.

[84] Acher CW, Wynn MM. Thoracoabdominal aortic aneurysm. How we do it. Cardiovasc Surg. 1999;7:593-596. DOI: 10.1016/s0967-2109(99)00037-x.

[85] Malouf JF, Chandrasekaran K, Orszulak TA. Mycotic aneurysms of the thoracic aorta: a diagnostic challenge. Am J Med. 2003;115:489-496. DOI: 10.1016/s0002-9343(03)00394-2.

[86] Sessa C, Farah I, Voirin L, Magne JL, Brion JP, Guidicelli H. Infected aneurysms of the infrarenal abdominal aorta: diagnostic criteria and therapeutic strategy. Ann Vasc Surg. 1997;11:453-463. DOI: 10.1007/s100169900075.

[87] Pasic M, Carrel T, Tönz M, Vogt P, von Segesser L, Turina M. Mycotic aneurysm of the abdominal aorta: extra-anatomic versus in situ reconstruction. Cardiovasc Surg. 1993;1:48-52.

[88] Clagett GP, Valentine RJ, Hagino RT. Autogenous aortoiliac/femoral reconstruction from superficial femoral-popliteal veins: feasibility and durability. J Vasc Surg. 1997;25:255-266. DOI: 10.1016/s0741-5214(97)70347-1.

[89] Modrall JG, Hocking JA, Timaran CH, Rosero EB, Arko FR 3rd, Valentine RJ, Clagett GP. Late incidence of chronic venous insufficiency after deep vein harvest. J Vasc Surg. 2007;46:520-525. DOI: 10.1016/j.jvs.2007.04.061.

[90] Brown KE, Heyer K, Rodriguez H, Eskandari MK, Pearce WH, Morasch MD. Arterial reconstruction with cryopreserved human allografts in the setting of infection: a single-center experience with midterm follow-up. J Vasc Surg. 2009;49:660-666. DOI: 10.1016/j.jvs.2008.10.026.

[91] Bisdas T, Wilhelmi M, Haverich A, Teebken OE. Cryopreserved arterial homografts vs silver-coated Dacron grafts for abdominal aortic infections with intraoperative evidence of microorganisms. J Vasc Surg. 2011;53:1274-1281. DOI: 10.1016/j.jvs.2010.11.052.

[92] Taylor LM Jr, Deitz DM, McConnell DB, Porter JM. Treatment of infected abdominal aneurysms by extraanatomic bypass, aneurysm excision, and drainage. Am J Surg. 1988;155:655-658. DOI: 10.1016/s0002-9610(88)80137-5.

[93] Lee CH, Hsieh HC, Ko PJ, Li HJ, Kao TC, Yu SY. In situ versus extra-anatomic reconstruction for primary infected infrarenal abdominal aortic aneurysms. J Vasc Surg. 2011;54:64-70. DOI: 10.1016/j.jvs.2010.12.032.

[94] Inoue H, Iguro Y, Ueno M, Yamamoto K. Extra-anatomic bypass operation for an infected aortic arch aneurysm with broad mediastinal abscess: a case report. Ann Vasc Dis. 2015;8:246-248. DOI: 10.3400/avd.cr.15-00009.

[95] Woon CY, Sebastian MG, Tay KH, Tan SG. Extra-anatomic revascularization and aortic exclusion for mycotic aneurysms of the infrarenal aorta and iliac arteries in an Asian population. Am J Surg. 2008;195:66-72. DOI: 10.1016/j.amjsurg.2007.01.032.

[96] Semba CP, Sakai T, Slonim SM, Razavi MK, Kee ST, Jorgensen MJ, Hagberg RC, Lee GK, Mitchell RS, Miller DC, Dake MD. Mycotic aneurysms of the thoracic aorta: repair with use of endovascular stent-grafts. J Vasc Interv Radiol. 1998;9:33-40. DOI: 10.1016/s1051-0443(98)70479-8.

[97] Jones KG, Bell RE, Sabharwal T, Aukett M, Reidy JF, Taylor PR. Treatment of mycotic aortic aneurysms with endoluminal grafts. Eur J Vasc Endovasc Surg. 2005;29:139-144. DOI: 10.1016/j.ejvs.2004.11.008.

[98] Clough RE, Black SA, Lyons OT, Zayed HA, Bell RE, Carrell T, Waltham M, Sabharwal T, Taylor PR. Is endovascular repair of mycotic aortic aneurysms a durable treatment option? Eur J Vasc Endovasc Surg. 2009;37:407-412. DOI: 10.1016/j.ejvs.2008.11.025.

[99] Chiesa R, Melissano G, Marrocco-Trischitta MM, Civilini E, Setacci F. Spinal cord ischemia after elective stent-graft repair of the thoracic aorta. J Vasc Surg. 2005;42:11-17. DOI: 10.1016/j.jvs.2005.04.016.

[100] Buth J, Harris PL, Hobo R, van Eps R, Cuypers P, Duijm L, Tielbeek X. Neurologic complications associated with endovascular repair of thoracic aortic pathology: incidence and risk factors. A study from the European Collaborators on Stent/Graft Techniques for Aortic Aneurysm Repair (EUROSTAR) registry. J Vasc Surg. 2007;46:1103-1110. DOI: 10.1016/j.jvs.2007.08.020.

[101] Ozsvath KJ, Roddy SP, Darling RC 3rd, Byrne J, Kreienberg PB, Choi D, Paty PS, Chang BB, Mehta M, Shah DM. Carotid-carotid crossover bypass: is it a durable procedure? J Vasc Surg. 2003;37:582-585. DOI: 10.1067/mva.2003.128.

[102] Cires G, Noll RE Jr, Albuquerque FC Jr, Tonnessen BH, Sternbergh WC 3rd. Endovascular debranching of the aortic arch during thoracic endograft repair. J Vasc Surg. 2011;53:1485-1491. DOI: 10.1016/j.jvs.2011.01.053.

[103] Ohrlander T, Sonesson B, Ivancev K, Resch T, Dias N, Malina M. The chimney graft: a technique for preserving or rescuing aortic branch vessels in stent-graft sealing zones. J Endovasc Ther. 2008;15:427-432. DOI: 10.1583/07-2315.1.

[104] Younes HK, Davies MG, Bismuth J, Naoum JJ, Peden EK, Reardon MJ, Lumsden AB. Hybrid thoracic endovascular aortic repair: pushing the envelope. J Vasc Surg. 2010;51:259-266. DOI: 10.1016/j.jvs.2009.09.043.

[105] Andersen ND, Williams JB, Hanna JM, Shah AA, McCann RL, Hughes GC. Results with an algorithmic approach to hybrid repair of the aortic arch. J Vasc Surg. 2013;57:655-667. DOI: 10.1016/j.jvs.2012.09.039.

[106] Heye S, Daenens K, Maleux G, Nevelsteen A. Stent-graft repair of a mycotic ascending aortic pseudoaneurysm. J Vasc Interv Radiol. 2006;17:1821-1825. DOI: 10.1097/01.RVI.0000244834.71601.65.

[107] Vaughan-Huxley E, Hamady MS, Metcalfe MJ, Adams B, Kashef E, Cheshire NJ, Bicknell CD. Endovascular repair of an acute, mycotic, ascending aortic pseudoaneurysm. Eur J Vasc Endovasc Surg. 2011;41:488-491. DOI: 10.1016/j.ejvs.2010.12.004.

[108] Quinney BE, Jordan W Jr. Branched endograft repair of mycotic ascending aortic aneurysm using the snorkel technique. Vasc Endovascular Surg. 2011;45:457-458. DOI: 10.1177/1538574411405222.

[109] Gelpi G, Cagnoni G, Vanelli P, Antona C. Endovascular repair of ascending aortic pseudoaneurysm in a high-risk patient. Interact Cardiovasc Thorac Surg. 2012;14:494-496. DOI: 10.1093/icvts/ivr134.

[110] Meerkin D, Yinnon AM, Munter RG, Shemesh O, Hiller N, Abraham AS. Salmonella mycotic aneurysm of the aortic arch: case report and review. Clin Infect Dis. 1995;21:523-528. DOI: 10.1093/clinids/21.3.523.

[111] Soravia-Dunand VA, Loo VG, Salit IE. Aortitis due to Salmonella: report of 10 cases and comprehensive review of the literature. Clin Infect Dis. 1999;29:862-868. DOI: 10.1086/520450.

[112] Weis-Müller BT, Rascanu C, Sagban A, Grabitz K, Godehardt E, Sandmann W. Single-center experience with open surgical treatment of 36 infected aneurysms of the thoracic, thoracoabdominal, and abdominal aorta. Ann Vasc Surg. 2011;25:1020-1025. DOI: 10.1016/j.avsg.2011.03.009.

[113] Hsu RB, Lin FY. Surgery for infected aneurysm of the aortic arch. J Thorac Cardiovasc Surg. 2007;134:1157-1162. DOI: 10.1016/j.jtcvs.2007.07.009.

[114] Hsu RB, Lin FY. Infected aneurysm of the thoracic aorta. J Vasc Surg. 2008;47:270-276. DOI: 10.1016/j.jvs.2007.10.017.

[115] Hsu RB, Chang CI, Chan CY, Wu IH. Infected aneurysms of the suprarenal abdominal aorta. J Vasc Surg. 2011;54:972-978. DOI: 10.1016/j.jvs.2011.04.024.

[116] Yu SY, Hsieh HC, Ko PJ, Huang YK, Chu JJ, Lee CH. Surgical outcome for mycotic aortic and iliac anuerysm. World J Surg. 2011;35:1671-1678. DOI: 10.1007/s00268-011-1104-9.

[117] Uchida N, Katayama A, Tamura K, Miwa S, Masatsugu K, Sueda T. In situ replacement for mycotic aneurysms on the thoracic and abdominal aorta using rifampicin-bonded grafting and omental pedicle grafting. Ann Thorac Surg. 2012;93:438-442. DOI: 10.1016/j.athoracsur.2011.07.050.

[118] Lin CH, Hsu RB. Primary infected aortic aneurysm: clinical presentation, pathogen, and outcome. Acta Cardiol Sin. 2014;30:514-521.

[119] Carrel T, Pasic M, Bino M, Turina M. Recurrent rupture of a mycotic ascending aortic aneurysm: a surgical and medical challenge. Eur J Cardiothorac Surg. 1992;6:158-160. DOI: 10.1016/1010-7940(92)90123-f.

[120] Risher WH, McFadden PM. Neisseria gonorrhoeae mycotic ascending aortic aneurysm. Ann Thorac Surg. 1994;57:748-750. DOI: 10.1016/0003-4975(94)90583-5.

[121] Kubota H, Endo H, Noma M, Tsuchiya H, Yoshimoto A, Takahashi Y, Inaba Y, Matsukura M, Sudo K. Equine pericardial roll graft replacement of infected pseudoaneurysm of the ascending aorta. J Cardiothorac Surg. 2012;7:54. DOI: 10.1186/1749-8090-7-54.

[122] Yano M, Hayase T, Furukawa K, Nakamura K. Mycotic pseudoaneurysm of the ascending aorta caused by *Escherichia coli*. Interact Cardiovasc Thorac Surg. 2013;16:81-83. DOI: 10.1093/icvts/ivs376.

[123] Behzadnia N, Ahmadi ZH, Mandegar MH, Salehi F, Sharif-Kashani B, Pourabdollah M, Ansari-Aval Z, Kianfar AA, Mirhosseini SM, Eiji M. Asymptomatic mycotic aneurysm of ascending aorta after heart transplantation: a case report. Transplant Proc. 2015;47:213-216. DOI: 10.1016/j.transproceed.2014.10.036.

[124] Patel HJ, Williams DM, Upchurch GR Jr, Dasika NL, Eliason JL, Deeb GM. Thoracic aortic endovascular repair for mycotic aneurysms and fistulas. J Vasc Surg. 2010;52:37S-40S. DOI: 10.1016/j.jvs.2010.06.139.

[125] Antoniou GA, Koutsias S, Antoniou SA, Georgiakakis A, Lazarides MK, Giannoukas AD.Outcome after endovascular stent graft repair of aortoenteric fistula: a systematic review. J Vasc Surg. 2009;49:782-789. DOI: 10.1016/j.jvs.2008.08.068.

[126] Chiesa R, Melissano G, Marone EM, Kahlberg A, Marrocco-Trischitta MM, Tshomba Y. Endovascular treatment of aortoesophageal and aortobronchial fistulae. J Vasc Surg. 2010;51:1195-1202. DOI: 10.1016/j.jvs.2009.10.130.

[127] Setacci C, de Donato G, Setacci F. Endografts for the treatment of aortic infection. Semin Vasc Surg. 2011;24:242-249. DOI: 10.1053/j.semvascsurg.2011.10.009.

[128] John R, Korula RJ, Lal N, Shukla V, Lalitha MK. Salmonellosis complicating aortic aneurysms. Int Angiol. 1994;13:177-180.

[129] Hsu RB, Tsay YG, Wang SS, Chu SH. Management of aortic aneurysm infected with Salmonella. Br J Surg. 2003;90:1080-1084. DOI: 10.1002/bjs.4170.

[130] Fernández Guerrero ML, Aguado JM, Arribas A, Lumbreras C, de Gorgolas M. The spectrum of cardiovascular infections due to Salmonella enterica: a review of clinical features and factors determining outcome. Medicine (Baltimore). 2004;83:123-38. DOI: 10.1097/01.md.0000125652.75260.cf.

[131] Hsu RB, Lin FY, Chen RJ, Hsueh PR, Wang SS. Antimicrobial drug resistance in salmonella-infected aortic aneurysms. Ann Thorac Surg. 2005;80:530-536. DOI: 10.1016/j.athoracsur.2005.02.046.

[132] Forbes TL, Harding GE. Endovascular repair of Salmonella-infected abdominal aortic aneurysms: a word of caution. J Vasc Surg. 2006;44:198-200. DOI: 10.1016/j.jvs.2006.03.002.

[133] Ohki S, Hirai H, Yasuhara K, Hatori K, Miki T, Obayashi T. Aortoiliac artery reconstruction using bilateral reversed superficial femoral veins for an infected abdominal aortic aneurysm. Ann Vasc Dis. 2016;9:70-72. DOI: 10.3400/avd.cr.15-00122.

[134] Landau JH, Nagpal AD, Chu MW. Autologous pericardial reconstruction of ruptured Salmonella mycotic aortic arch aneurysm. Can J Cardiol. 2016;32:136.e1-e3. DOI: 10.1016/j.cjca.2015.08.013.

[135] Robinson JA, Johansen K. Aortic sepsis: is there a role for in situ graft reconstruction? J Vasc Surg. 1991;13:677-682. DOI: 10.1016/0741-5214(91)90353-v.

[136] Gupta AK, Bandyk DF, Johnson BL. In situ repair of mycotic abdominal aortic aneurysms with rifampicin-bonded gelatin-impregnated Dacron grafts: a preliminary case report. J Vasc Surg. 1996;24:472-476. DOI: 10.1016/s0741-5214(96)70204-5.

[137] Jia X, Dong YF, Liu XP, Xiong J, Zhang HP, Guo W. Open and endovascular repair of primary mycotic aortic aneurysms: a 10-year single-center experience. J Endovasc Ther. 2013;20:305-310. DOI: 10.1583/13-4222MR.1.

Chapter 10

Computational Fluid Dynamics of Blood Flow in the Abdominal Aorta Post "Chimney" Endovascular Aneurysm Repair (ChEVAR)

Hila Ben Gur, Moses Brand, Gábor Kósa and Saar Golan

Additional information is available at the end of the chapter

http://dx.doi.org/10.5772/64611

Abstract

Abdominal aortic aneurysms (AAAs) are a significant cause of death in the Western world. Endovascular aneurysm repair (EVAR) is becoming the prevalently used procedure to repair AAAs (versus the traditional approach of open surgery). In cases of infrarenal AAAs, there is a risk of the renal arteries being blocked by the stent graft (SG) inserted to repair the aneurysm. In these cases, two additional SGs termed"chimney" stent grafts (CSGs) are inserted into the renal arteries in parallel with the main SG to exclude this hazard. In this study, the hemodynamics of an infrarenal AAA endovascularly repaired by a system of SGs using the "chimney" technique is investigated. Two AAA models are analyzed using computational fluid dynamics (CFD, Ansys Fluent)—a healthy abdominal aorta and an abdominal aorta post"chimney" endovascular aneurysm repair (ChEVAR) with a CSG inserted into each renal artery in parallel with the aortic SG. Results indicate that CSGs induce stagnation zones downstream the renal arteries yet mild and confined overall flow and wall shear stress (WSS) modifications. The flow regime remains principally laminar. The study findings indicate the limited hemodynamic modifications of the ChEVAR procedure and thus further support its merit.

Keywords: abdominal aortic aneurysm (AAA), "chimney" endovascular aneurysm repair (ChEVAR), chimney stent graft (CSG), computational fluid dynamics (CFD), hemodynamics, wall shear stress (WSS)

1. Introduction

Aortic aneurysms (AAs) affect 5–7% of older Americans [1], causing about 15,000 deaths each year, of which 9000 are caused by abdominal aortic aneurysms (AAAs) [1, 2]. Risk of rupture within 1 year for patients with an initial AAA diameter of 5.5–5.9 cm is 9.4% and rises with increase in initial diameter [3]. The most common location of aortic aneurysm formation is the infrarenal section [4].

The traditional method of aneurysm repair is open surgery, in which a large incision in the patient's abdomen facilitates access to the aneurysm site. In recent years, increasingly a number of aneurysms are repaired endovascularly, excluding the aneurysm using stent grafts (SGs) delivered to its site via the arterial system in a minimally invasive procedure. Typically, small incisions in the groin are created in order to provide access to the repair site using the femoral arteries as entry points. Following SG implantation, the aneurysm sac is sealed and blood subsequently flows through the new artificial conduit replacing the previously bulging section of the aorta.

Successful endovascular repair necessitates addressing the specific morphologies of the aneurysm and its surrounding blood vessels. Aneurysms with short proximal (close to the heart) necks account for about 15% of all AAAs [5]. These require the physician performing the procedure to be very accurate when choosing the location of graft deployment. An aneurysm located near a visceral artery ostium is even more challenging to repair endovascularly. Here, the main undertaking is to achieve an adequate seal using the SG while keeping the aortic branches unobstructed [6]. Innovative solutions for this type of predicament include the fenestrated SG (FSG) system. FSGs are custom tailored to the individual morphology of each patient and required months of preparation ahead of the actual procedure [7].

In critical cases where the patient condition does not allow to wait several months for a custom SG system to be manufactured, a novel solution is recently being employed using off-the-shelf SGs. This solution is an endovascular surgical procedure termed the"chimney" technique. In"chimney" endovascular aneurysm repair (ChEVAR), one or more tubular covered stents ("chimneys") are implanted inside the visceral arteries in parallel with the main aortic SG that excludes the aneurysm sac. These covered stents facilitate proper blood flow to arteries that would otherwise be blocked by the main aortic SG. A common case of repair with the"chimney" technique involves proximity of the aneurysm to the two renal arteries (**Figure 1**). In this case, in order to preserve blood flow to the kidneys, a chimney stent graft (CSG) is inserted into each renal artery.

In this study, we investigate the hemodynamics in the abdominal aorta post-ChEVAR and compare it with a healthy abdominal aorta (**Figures 1** and **2**).

Computational fluid dynamics (CFD, ANSYS Fluent package) simulations of pulsatile blood flow during the cardiac cycle are employed. An idealized anatomy of the abdominal aorta is assumed based on averaged measurements taken from cadaver specimens and patient angiograms [8].

The effects CSGs have on abdominal aortic velocity and wall shear stress (WSS) fields are analyzed by evaluating blood flow patterns and regimes.

http://dx.doi.org/10.5772/64611

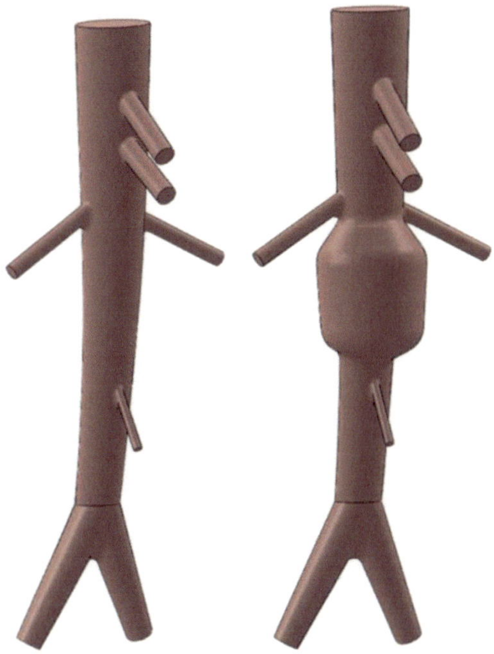

Figure 1. Left: healthy abdominal aorta model. Right: infrarenal aneurysmatic aorta.

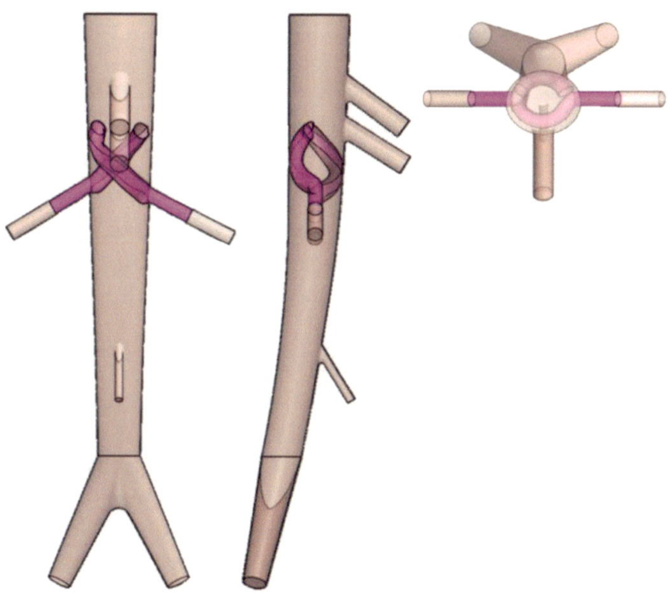

Figure 2. Model of the abdominal aorta post-ChEVAR (aneurysm fully replaced by SG). Left to right: front, side, and top views, respectively. Chimney SGs are highlighted pink.

2. Methodology

2.1. Governing equations

The governing equations for blood flow in the abdominal aorta are the Navier-Stokes Eq. (1) and the continuity Eq. (2) for an incompressible fluid:

$$\rho \partial v/\partial t + \rho(v \cdot \nabla)v - \mu \Delta v + \nabla\ P = 0 \tag{1}$$

$$\nabla\ \cdot v = 0 \tag{2}$$

where v, ρ, μ, and P denote the fluid velocity, density, dynamic viscosity (discussed in detail below), and the pressure field experienced by the fluid, respectively. Blood density is assumed as 1045 kg/m^3 [9]. ∇, $\nabla\cdot$, and ∇ denote the divergence, gradient, and Laplace operators, respectively.

2.2. Anatomical model

Figure 1 presents views of the three-dimensional (3D) model used for analysis of the idealized healthy abdominal aorta. The model is based on angiograms and pressurized cadaver specimens measurements [8]. This model accounts for the elliptical cross section and tapering of the abdominal aorta as it gives off the main arterial branches. It also includes the slight curvature toward the posterior wall. The seven main arterial branches are included: celiac trunk, superior mesenteric artery, left and right renal arteries, inferior mesenteric artery, and the left and right iliac arteries.

The model of the abdominal aorta post-ChEVAR is based on the healthy model. Modifications made account for the renal CSGs. The bulging part of the abdominal aorta is assumed to be completely replaced by the aortic SG and is not included in the analysis. The renal CSG is a covered tubular stent originally used for applications like femoral vascular access. In the"chimney" technique, CSGs are used to ensure blood flow into the renal arteries in cases where standard endovascular aneurysm repair (EVAR) might block the blood flow to these arteries. In this study, the CSGs are modeled as long tube-like structures having smooth inner and outer surfaces. The wall thickness of the CSGs is 0.1 mm, and its free diameter is 15–20% larger than the renal artery diameter. Here, a covered stent with a diameter of 7 mm is used [10, 11]. These dimensions are in compliance with common endograft dimensions in ChEVAR procedures. The three-dimensional shape of the renal CSGs after deployment is helical-like [12], and maintains an outline that does not block any of the major branching arteries.

The deployed CSG is in contact with different components along its length. It is restricted by the renal artery segment and then by the mixed contact area region where the CSG is confined by both the aorta wall and the main aortic SG. Each CSG ends in a segment that protrudes upstream from the aortic SG and into the main aortic duct (10 mm). At each of these segments, the CSG cross section is a little different as it morphs from a circle to a"flattened" elliptical shape and then to a larger circle [13]. These different cross sections are included in the numerical models. The CSG models also incorporate their helical-like nature [12].

http://dx.doi.org/10.5772/64611

Additional assumptions made in the study include rigid (nonflexible) walls, neglecting plaque and thrombus existence, and assuming postdeployment geometry only.

2.3. Numerical model

Blood flow behavior in the abdominal aorta along the cardiac cycle is considered to be predominantly laminar [14]. Thus, a laminar CFD solver is employed.

Literature demonstrates that flow characteristics, e.g., WSS, differ by as much as 30% between the distensible and rigid blood vessel models [15]. However, overall flow traits remain similar [16]. Therefore, rigid wall approximation is sufficient for a comparative study. The domain wall boundary conditions have no slip/penetration. The inlet BC is a pulsatile velocity function adapted from a flow rate waveform of an abdominal aorta during rest [17]. This waveform (**Figure 3**) was transformed into a Fourier series and then modified to represent the corresponding average velocity. The spatial distribution of the inlet velocity is approximated as a parabolic profile distributed over the elliptical inlet, and perpendicular to it [15, 18–20]. The seven domain outlets present constant flow ratios with the inlet throughout the cardiac cycle–celiac trunk—21%, superior mesenteric artery—15%, left and right renal arteries—15% each, inferior mesenteric artery—4%, and the left and right iliac arteries—15% each [8]. ANSYS Fluent CFD package is used for the analysis.

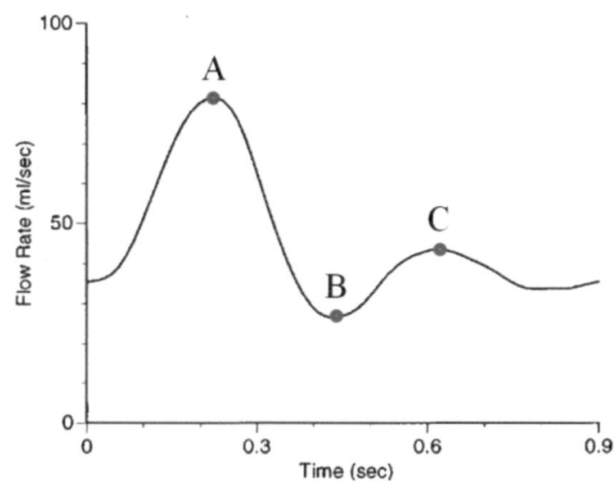

Figure 3. Inlet flow rate waveform (representing a single cycle). A: peak systole, B: start of diastole, and C: peak diastole [17].

2.4. Numerical discretization

The analysis uses second-order discretization schemes: in space, the least squares cell based for the gradient and the upwind for the momentum and in time the implicit. The spatial domain of the post-ChEVAR abdominal aorta is discretized using 2 million cells (**Figure 4**). Most cells are polyhedral, except prismatic cells used near wall regions to accommodate for the large gradients in these areas. The domain is discretized into tetrahedral elements in the Meshing module of the ANSYS software package and then converted into polyhedral elements in the Fluent module. The cycle is discretized into 400 time steps. The convergence criterion is a scaled residuals value of 10^{-4}. Periodic convergence is achieved in the third cardiac cycle. The numerical parameters used for the healthy aorta model are similar (**Figure 5**).

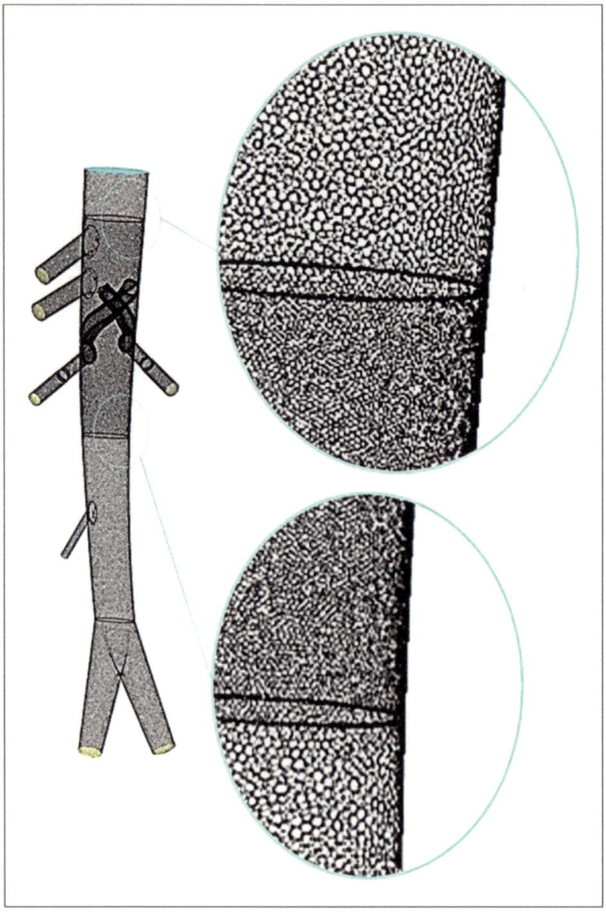

Figure 4. Post-ChEVAR model. Left: angled view. Right: close up of mesh transition zones (light blue ellipses).

2.5. Viscosity constitutive model

We studied two viscosity models—the Newtonian approximation and the Carreau constitutive law for shear-thinning fluids [9]. The Newtonian approximation assumes constant blood viscosity while the Carreau model accounts for the strain rate (**Table 1**):

$$\mu(\dot{\gamma}) = \mu_{\infty} + (\mu_0 - \mu_{\infty})\,(1 + \lambda^2 \dot{\gamma}^2)^{0.5(n-1)} \tag{3}$$

where $\dot{\gamma}$ represents the scalar flow shear rate and μ_8 and μ_0 represent the viscosities for infinitely large and zero strain rates, respectively. λ and n are fluid-specific time constant and power index, respectively (**Table 1**). The Newtonian viscosity is taken as the viscosity of blood under infinite shear rate, as commonly assumed for blood flow in large arteries such as the aorta [14, 21].

http://dx.doi.org/10.5772/64611

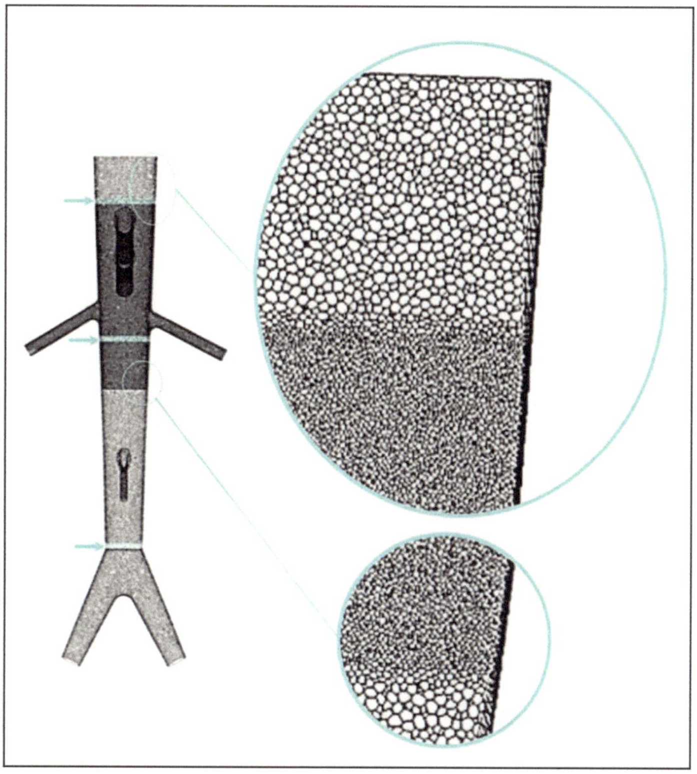

Figure 5. Healthy aorta model. Left: wall surfaces evaluated in order to compare the Newtonian and Carreau constitutive models. Top to bottom (in light blue): supra-celiac, infrarenal, and supra-bifurcation cross sections. Right: close up of mesh transition zones (light blue ellipses).

Newtonian viscosity	Carreau viscosity parameters
$\mu = 0.0033$ Pa·s	$\lambda = 1$ s
	$n = 0.4$
	$\mu_0 = 0.016$ Pa·s
	$\mu_8 = 0.0033$ Pa·s

Table 1. Fluid properties for the Newtonian and Carreau blood viscosity models [9].

CFD simulations were performed for the healthy abdominal aorta using both the Newtonian and Carreau viscosity models. Three wall locations were used in order to compare the WSS behaviors of the two models (**Figure 5**). The time-resolved WSSs (axial-Y components) at these locations display different systolic and diastolic peak values (**Figure 6**). The Newtonian model consistently presents peak values lower than the Carreau model at all three locations. Additionally, the systolic phases at the infrarenal height have opposite sign derivatives during (0.15–0.25) $\cdot t/T$. The two models generate significantly different mean WSS values—14–20% (**Table 2**). Interestingly, the Carreau model consistently predicts higher absolute value shear stresses. The flows predicted using the two models also exhibit different patterns. The flow consistently presents more disturbed designs when employing the Newtonian model (**Figures 7–9**).

Since the discrepancies between the results of both models are not negligible, best practice is to choose the viscosity model that better describes blood behavior–the Carreau model.

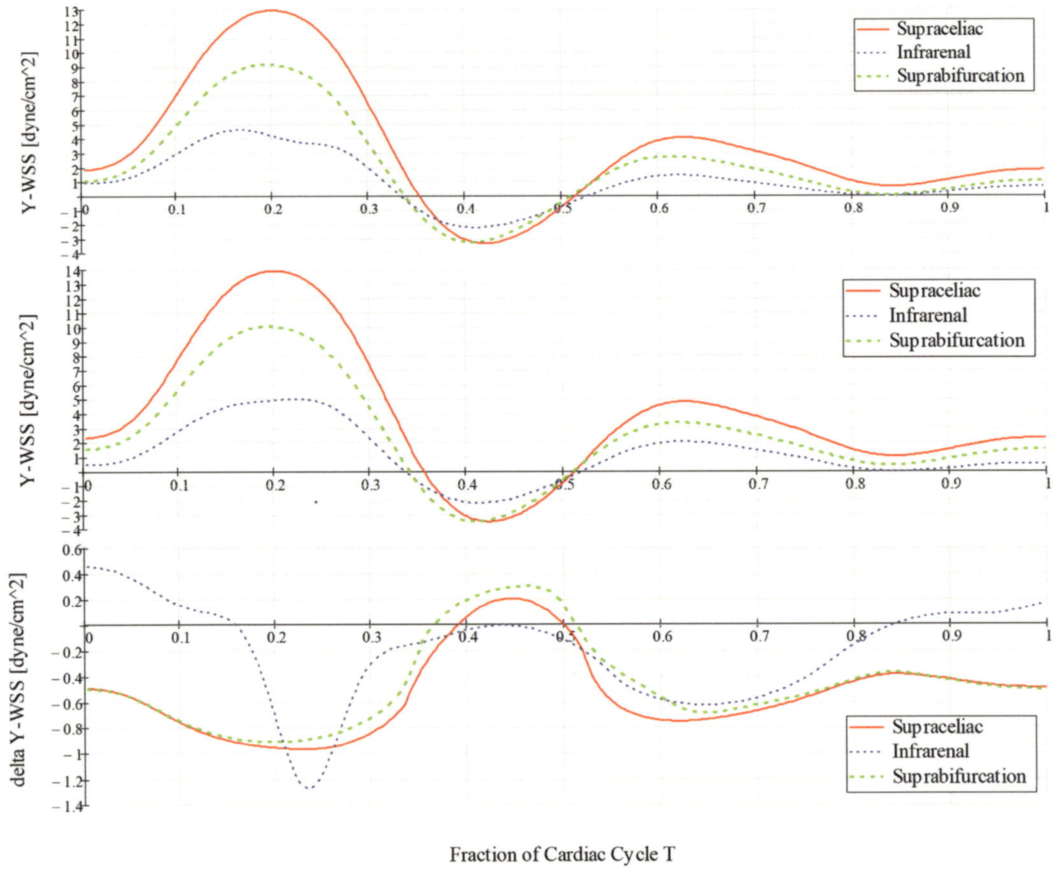

Figure 6. Time-resolved WSS (axial-Y components) curves. Top: Newtonian viscosity model, middle: Carreau viscosity model, bottom: difference between the Newtonian and Carreau models.

WSS (dyne/cm²)	Supra-celiac	Infrarenal	Supra-bifurcation
Newtonian	-3.29	-0.888	-1.98
Carreau	-3.832	-1.106	-2.453
Difference (%)	-14	-20	-19

Table 2. Mean WSS (axial component) for the Newtonian and Carreau viscosity models.

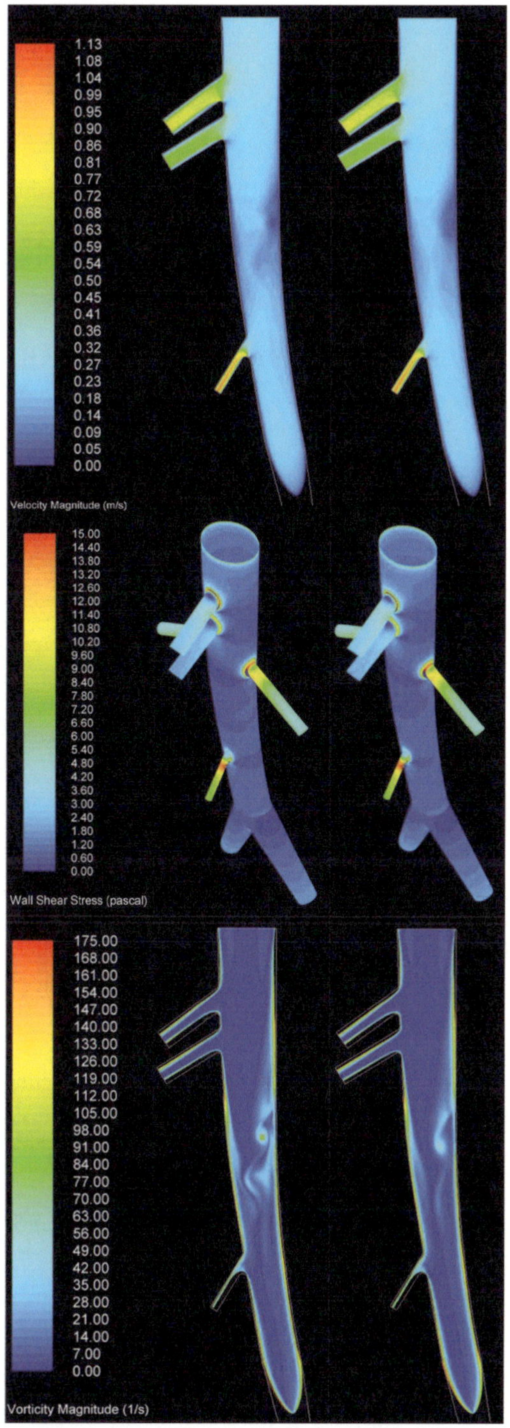

Figure 7. Contour plots of the hemodynamic conditions at peak systole. Left: Newtonian model. Right: Carreau model. Top row: velocity magnitude. Middle row: WSS magnitude. Bottom row: vorticity magnitude.

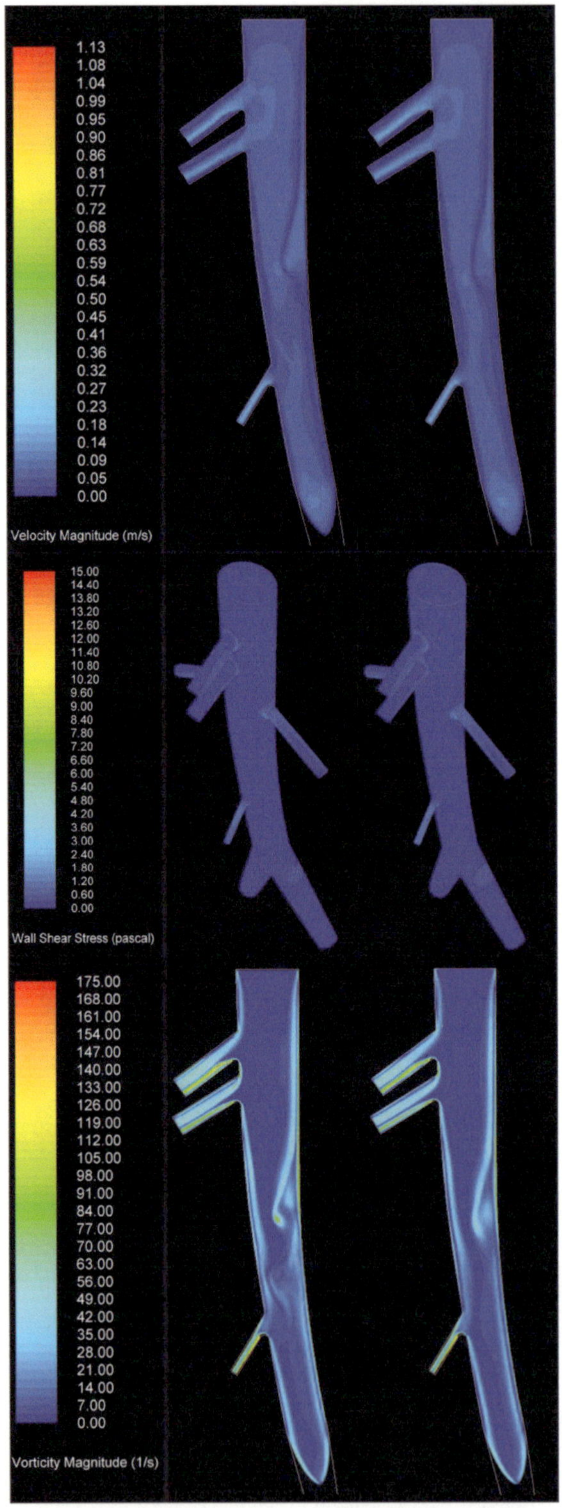

Figure 8. Contour plots of the hemodynamic conditions at the start of diastole. Left: Newtonian model. Right: Carreau model. Top row: velocity magnitude. Middle row: WSS magnitude. Bottom row: vorticity magnitude.

http://dx.doi.org/10.5772/64611

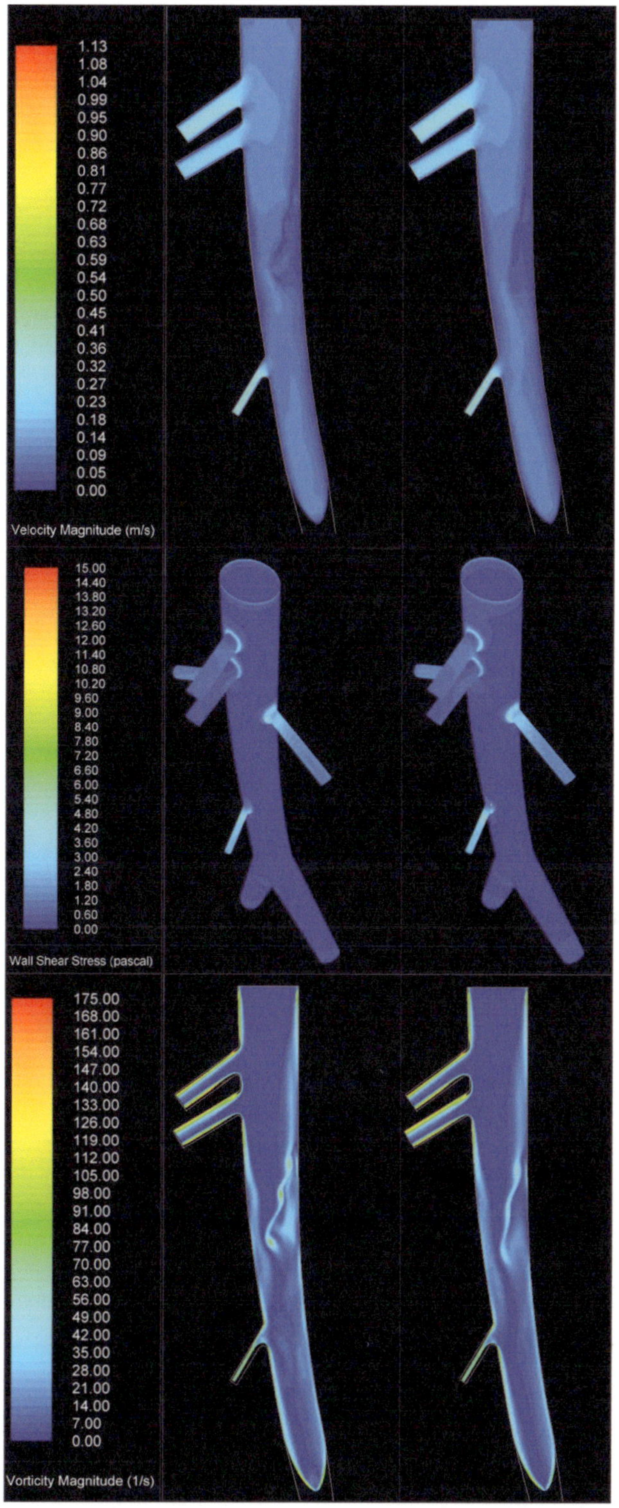

Figure 9. Contour plots of the hemodynamic conditions at peak diastole. Left: Newtonian model. Right: Carreau model. Top row: velocity magnitude. Middle row: WSS magnitude. Bottom row: vorticity magnitude.

3. Results

3.1. Validation

WSS for the healthy aorta (supra-celiac section) was compared with experimental data available in the literature (**Table 3**) [22]. The temporal minimum, maximum, and average WSS values of each mesh cell at the supra-celiac ring of **Figure 10** were extracted from a full cardiac cycle. The spatial average of each of these parameters along the ring circumference was calculated and tabulated. Pulse WSS is the difference between the maximum and minimum WSSs for each element (also spatially averaged along the circumference). The differences evident in this comparison indicate that the numerical results are in reasonable agreement with the experimental data (**Table 3**).

WSS (Pa)	Minimum	Maximum	Average	Pulse
Experiment	-0.45	0.87	0.13	1.32
Numerical model	-0.48	0.99	0.19	1.47
Difference (%)	6	14	44	12

Table 3. WSS numerical validation results (axial-Y component), supra-celiac region.

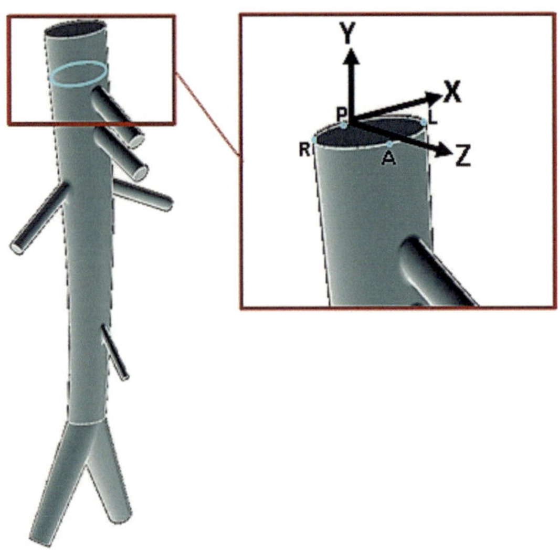

Figure 10. Left: supra-celiac WSS comparison contour (highlighted blue). Right: coordinate system and regions of interest: A—anterior, P—posterior, R—right, L—left.

3.2. Flow patterns

Stagnant regions are formed in the post-ChEVAR aorta downstream from and in close proximity to the CSGs. These regions persist throughout the cardiac cycle, as demonstrated by velocity

http://dx.doi.org/10.5772/64611

contours plotted at the peak of the systole and at the start of the diastole—see **Figures 11** and **12**. These stagnant regions are not present in the healthy model—see **Figures 13** and **14**.

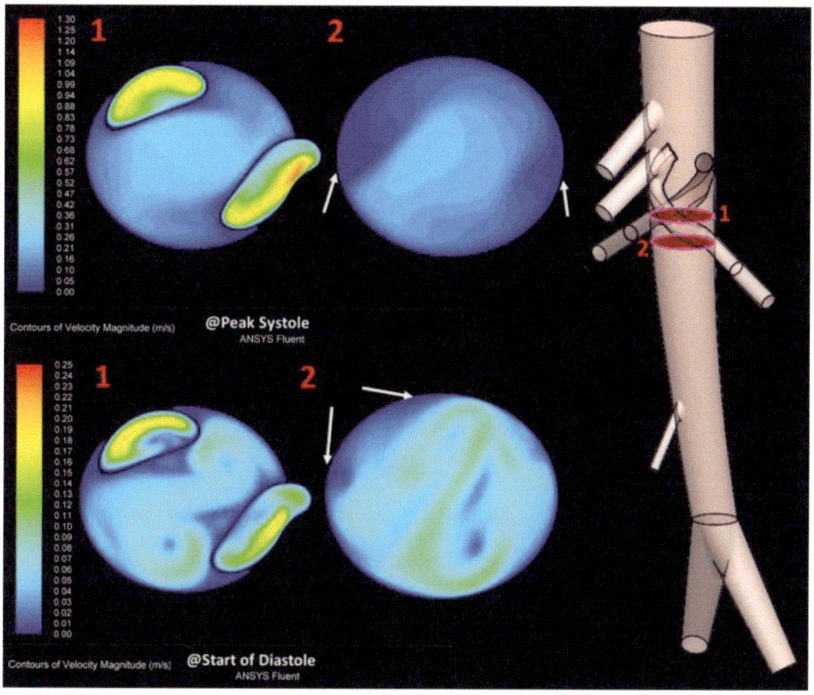

Figure 11. Contour plots of blood velocity for the post-ChEVAR model at two horizontal sections below the CSGs (marked red on the right). Top row: peak systole. Bottom row: start of diastole. Arrows: stagnant regions.

The healthy model portrays recirculation and stagnation zones along the infrarenal segment of the posterior wall of the abdominal aortic duct (**Figure 14**). This is evident in the form of closed single-colored patches of low velocity in the **start of the diastole** and the **peak of the diastole**, and less distinctly in the **peak of the systole**. Similar patterns do not appear at this region for the post-ChEVAR model (**Figure 12**).

Several low velocity patches are present downstream from the CSGs for the post-ChEVAR model in the **start of the diastole** and **the peak of the diastole**. In the **start of the diastole**, disorganized streaks and variation in velocity values (contour colors) appear in the renal arteries for the post-ChEVAR model. Stagnation zones radially surround the CSG cross sections for the post-ChEVAR model in all three critical instants A–C of **Figure 3** (**Figures 11** and **12**). In the **peak of the systole** and **the peak of the diastole** the stagnation zones are somewhat elongated in the downstream direction from the CSGs and along the aortic wall.

Figure 15 displays vector plots of the blood velocity in the beginning of the diastole along the flow direction. The flow patterns for the two models are similar for the section ranging from the inlet and downstream roughly to the location of the celiac trunk and in the segment ranging from the inferior mesenteric artery downstream to the iliac arteries outlets. This holds for

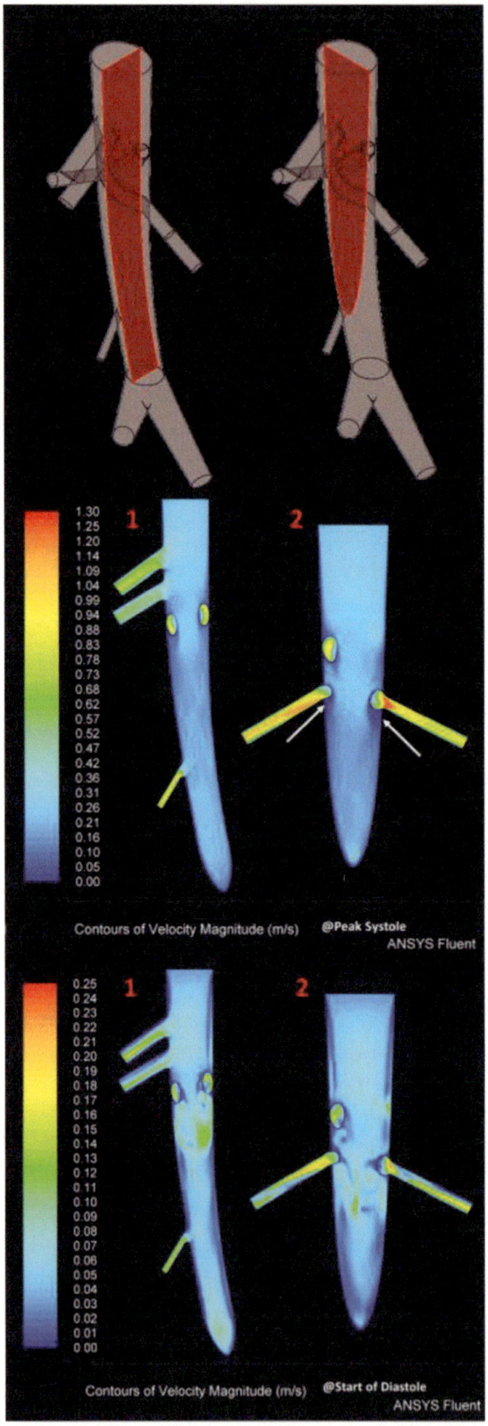

Figure 12. Contour plots of blood velocity for the post ChEVAR model at two vertical sections (marked red at the top row). Middle row: peak systole. Bottom row: start of diastole.

all three critical instants A–C of **Figure 3**. Several discrepancies are apparent in the middle segment, most notably in the infrarenal region. Here, reverse (retro) flow occurs near the walls in the post-ChEVAR model while in the healthy model these flows take place generally about the centerline (with most flow oriented forward). Additionally, the post-ChEVAR model exhibits somewhat disorganized forward flow in this area while the flow in the healthy model is more structured. Lastly, the velocity profiles along both renal arteries are notably skewed in the post-ChEVAR model compared with the healthy model.

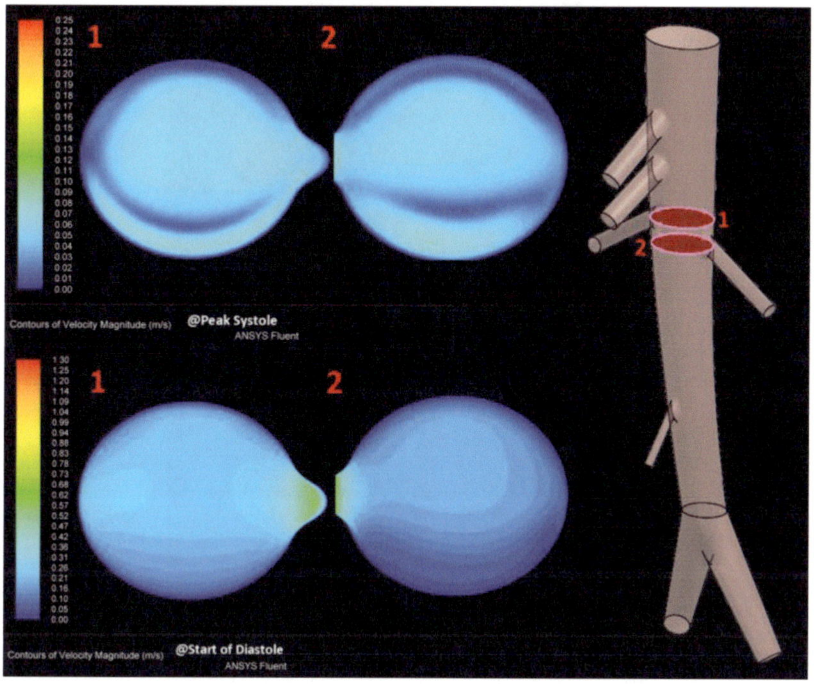

Figure 13. Contour plots of blood velocity for the healthy model at two horizontal sections below the CSGs position (marked red on the right, same locations as in **Figure 11**). Top row: peak systole. Bottom row: start of diastole.

Figure 16 displays contours of the WSS magnitude at the walls for the two models in the three critical instants A–C of **Figure 3**—peak systole, beginning of diastole, and peak diastole. The post-ChEVAR model exhibits low WSS at the CSGs and aortic wall contact zones. Close to these low WSS areas, slightly higher WSS regions in the shape of disorganized patches are present in the peak of the systole and the start of the diastole. Similar regions are present but take the shape of circumferential bands in the peak of the diastole.

For two segments of the aorta, the WSS distributions for the post-ChEVAR model are very similar to those for the healthy model in all three critical instances. These are the segments ranging from the inlet to just downstream of the celiac artery ostium and from roughly mid length between the left renal artery ostium and the inferior mesenteric artery ostium to just downstream of the iliac arteries outlets.

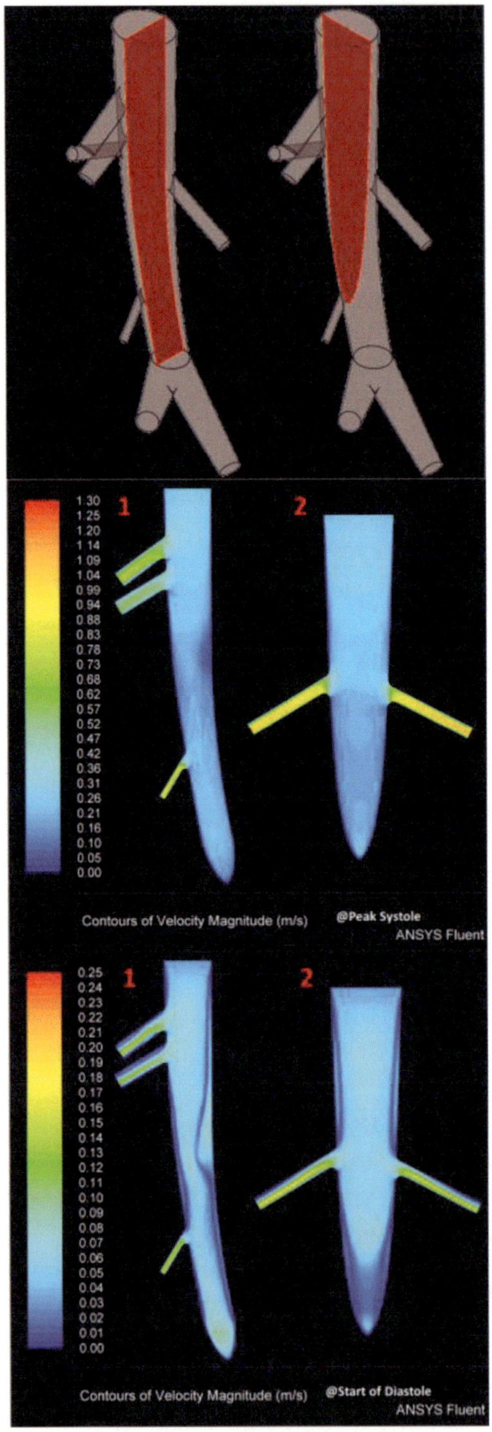

Figure 14. Contour plots of blood velocity for the healthy model at two vertical sections (marked red at the top row, same locations as in **Figure 12**). Middle row: peak systole. Bottom row: start of diastole.

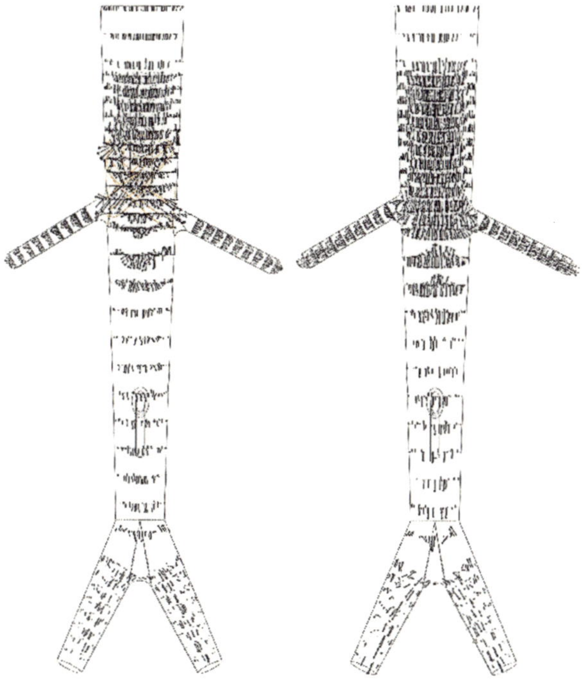

Figure 15. Vector plots of blood velocity in the beginning of the diastole. Left: post-ChEVAR model. Right: healthy model.

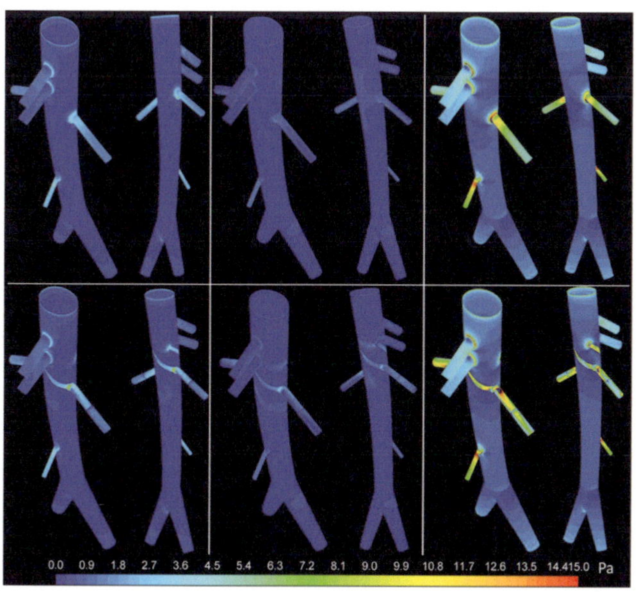

Figure 16. Contours of WSS magnitude at the walls—rotated anterior and posterior views. Top row: healthy model. Bottom row: post-ChEVAR model. Right to left columns: peak systole, start of diastole, and peak diastole.

3.3. Flow regime

Figure 17 illustrates key locations of interest for which WSSs were evaluated throughout the cardiac cycle. The axial-Y components of these WSSs are plotted along the various sides of the post-ChEVAR aorta (right, left, anterior, and posterior) throughout the cardiac cycle in **Figures 18–20**. **Figure 21** illustrates the axial component of the velocity along the centerline for the post-ChEVAR aorta throughout the cardiac cycle.

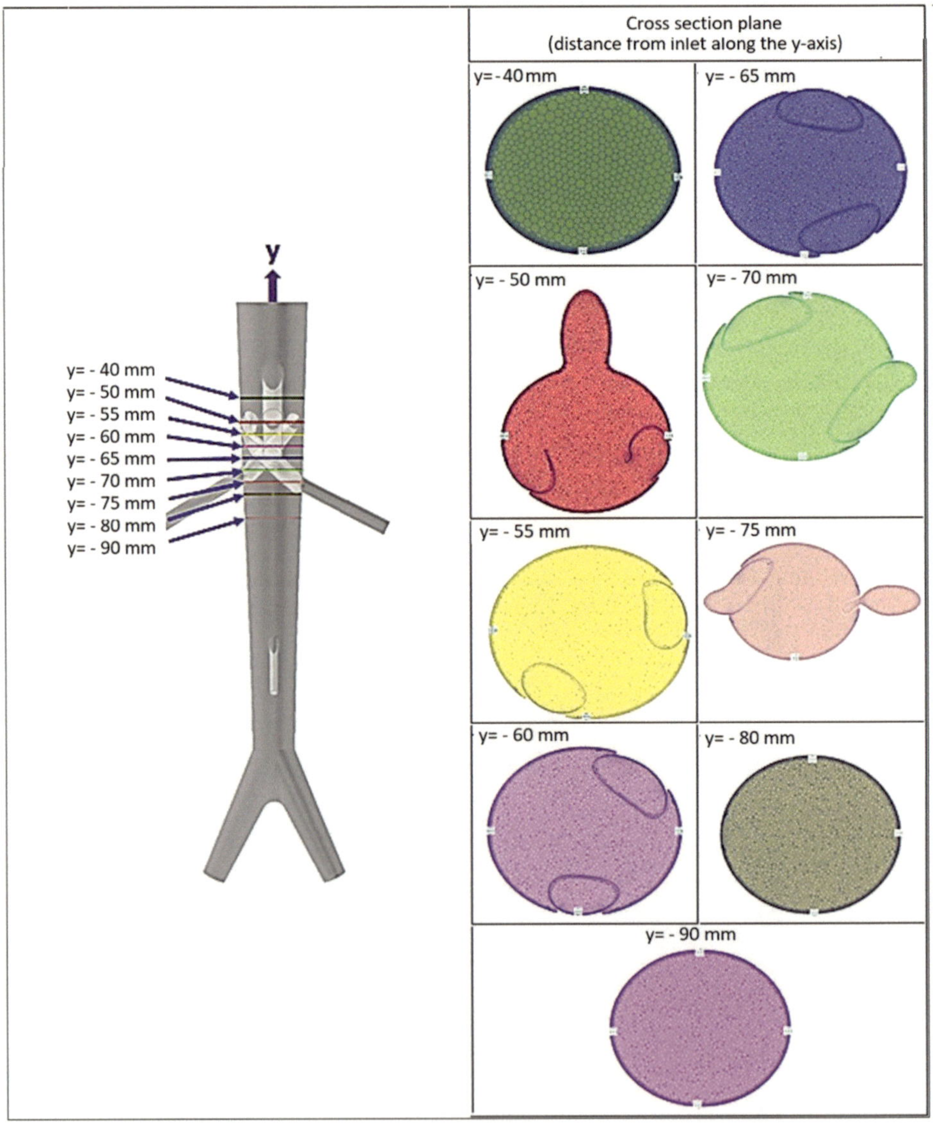

Figure 17. The different horizontal planes evaluated for WSSs for the post-ChEVAR model. Left: section planes and their distances from the inlet. Right: the specific points of WSS evaluation at each plane (marked by a dot sign).

http://dx.doi.org/10.5772/64611

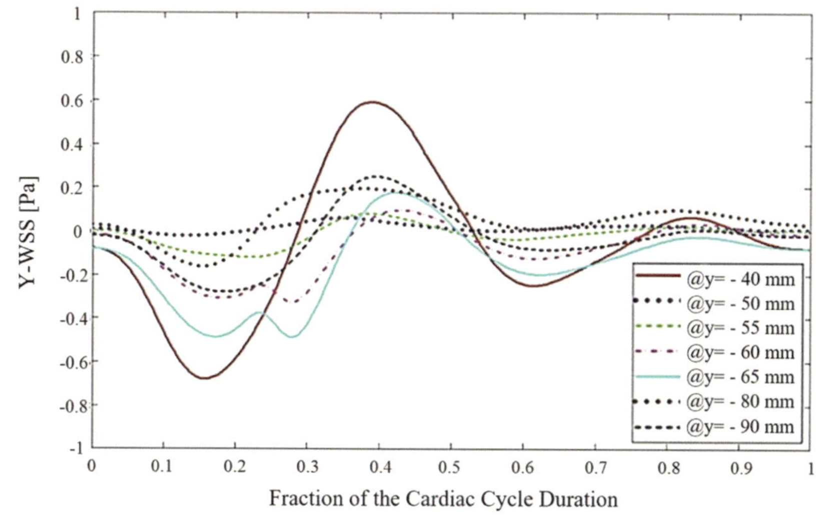

Figure 18. Axial component of the WSS along the right side of the post-ChEVAR aorta throughout the cardiac cycle.

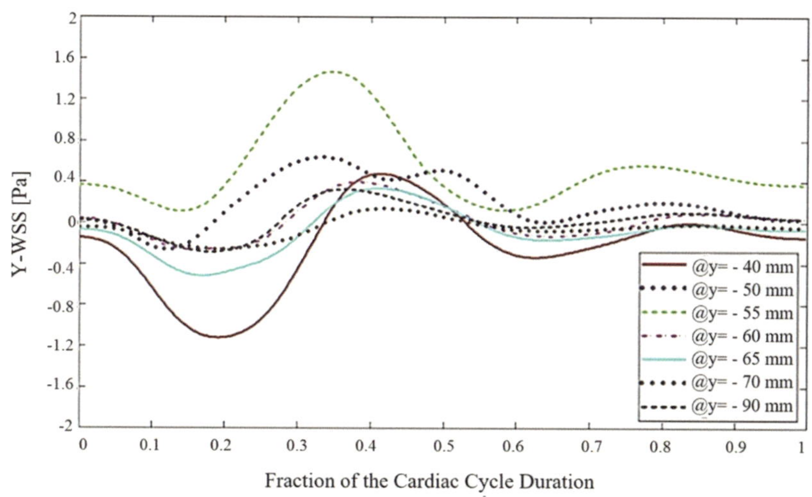

Figure 19. Axial component of the WSS along the left side of the post-ChEVAR aorta throughut the cardiac cycle.

WSSs and velocity patterns follow the inlet flow waveform. There are no high frequency components present. When an inlet flow waveform is free of high frequency components yet locations inside the control volume present velocity/WSS waveforms having high frequency noise, the flow is typically transitional [23]. Here, however, all waveforms are free of high frequency components, thus indicating a laminar flow regime [23]. Therefore, the flow in the post-ChEVAR abdominal aorta is expected to be principally laminar.

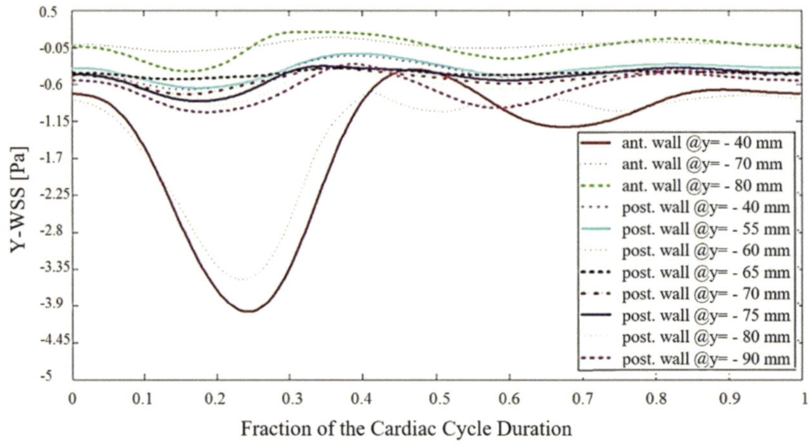

Figure 20. Axial component of the WSS along the anterior/posterior of the post-ChEVAR aorta throughout the cardiac cycle.

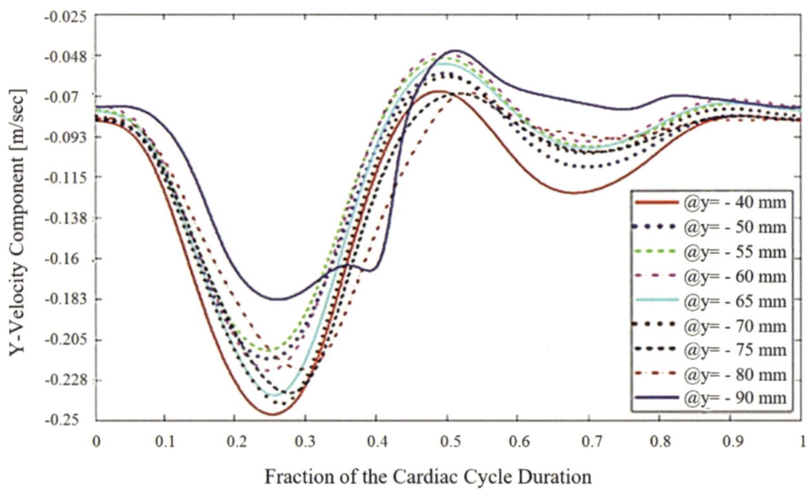

Figure 21. Axial component of the velocity along the centerline of the post-ChEVAR aorta throughout the cardiac cycle.

4. Discussion

This study sets out to determine the hemodynamic effects in the abdominal aorta as caused by CSGs placed in the renal arteries (as part of ChEVAR repair of infrarenal AAAs). A healthy aorta is employed as a baseline (control) for comparative study. Blood flow in the aorta is mostly adversely affected in the renal arteries region. This is expected since the CSGs constitute a substantial disturbance to the flow that does not exist in healthy abdominal aortas. Their presence induces stagnant velocity regions downstream from the renal arteries throughout the cardiac cycle that might promote thrombosis and inflammation.

Nevertheless, the negative effects of the ChEVAR repair appear relatively mild and are generally localized and confined to the CSGs' vicinity. The velocity fields further downstream for both models are nearly identical. The velocity fields' similarity holds for the upstream segment comprising the inlet as well. **Figure 15**—the vector plots of blood velocity—further supports the overall confined segmental nature of the ChEVAR technique.

The WSS field for the post-ChEVAR model exhibits irregularly shaped patches in the CSGs vicinity (**Figure 16**). In contrast, the WSS field for the healthy model is relatively uniform in this respective region, particularly in the peak of the systole and the beginning of the diastole. Nevertheless, as with the case of the velocity, the WSS fields for the post-ChEVAR model and for the healthy model are very similar downstream from the inferior mesenteric artery and from the inlet to slightly upstream from the CSGs. This again supports the overall confined nature of the ChEVAR technique.

The temporal behavior of the flow field and WSSs for the post-ChEVAR model presents no high frequency oscillations/components and appears to follow the inlet waveform. This indicates lack of turbulent or transitional flow and points toward a predominantly laminar flow regime. Thus, supporting yet again the overall confined nature of the CSG presence.

Overall, we conclude that CSGs are expected to induce localized effects in the hemodynamics of the abdominal aorta, mostly confined to the pararenal segment. This result supports the merit of the ChEVAR technique.

5. Conclusions

CSGs presence in the abdominal aorta introduces blood flow and WSSs patterns variations. In particular, the formation of stagnant regions downstream from the CSGs throughout the cardiac cycle, potentially contributing to thrombosis [24]. Nevertheless, in general, the flow field and WSSs appear to remain nearly unaffected in adjacent segments upstream and downstream from the CSGs site. The effects of the CSGs seem to extend about 1 cm upstream and to the approximate location of the inferior mesenteric artery ostium downstream. Furthermore, the CSGs do not appear to shift the flow regime to transitional or turbulent [23]. This suggests that the changes induced by CSGs are limited and confined in their nature, thus supporting the ChEVAR technique merit.

The zone most prone to atherosclerosis, thrombus formation, and other maladies appears to be the infrarenal section of the posterior wall of the abdominal aorta. These diseases are mechanistically linked to low and oscillating WSS [17]. As expected, the post-ChEVAR model is more adversely affected by these phenomena than the healthy model. These results mean that CSGs presence in infrarenal AAAs might function as a minor comorbidity factor in the future health of post-ChEVAR patients.

Our findings are in good agreement with data indicating a relatively high success rate for ChEVAR procedures performed in recent years, evident both in short- and long-term patient follow ups [25].

Author details

Hila Ben Gur[1], Moses Brand[2]*, Gábor Kósa[1] and Saar Golan[2, 3]

*Address all correspondence to: mosheb@ariel.ac.il

1 School of Mechanical Engineering, Faculty of Engineering, Tel Aviv University, Tel Aviv, Israel

2 Department of Mechanical Engineering & Mechatronics, Faculty of Engineering, Ariel University, Ariel, Israel

3 Department of Chemical Engineering, Faculty of Engineering, Ariel University, Ariel, Israel

References

[1] A. S. Les, S. C. Shadden, C. A. Figueroa, J. M. Park, M. M. Tedesco, R. J. Herfkens, R. L. Dalman, and C. A. Taylor, "Quantification of hemodynamics in abdominal aortic aneurysms during rest and exercise using magnetic resonance imaging and computational fluid dynamics," *Ann. Biomed. Eng.*, vol. 38, no. 4, pp. 1288–1313, 2010.

[2] C. Fleming, E. P. Whitlock, T. L. Beil, and F. A. Lederle, "Screening for abdominal aortic aneurysm: a best-evidence systematic review for the U.S. preventive services task force," *Ann. Intern. Med.*, vol. 142, no. 3, pp. 203–213, 2005.

[3] F. A. Lederle, G. R. Johnson, S. E. Wilson, D. J. Ballard, W. D. Jordan, J. Blebea, F. N. Littooy, J. A. Freischlag, D. Bandyk, J. H. Rapp, and A. A. Salam, "Rupture rate of large abdominal aortic aneurysms in patients refusing or unfit for elective repair," *JAMA*, vol. 287, no. 22, pp. 2968–2972, 2002.

[4] D.C. Guo, C. L. Papke, R. He, and D. M. Milewicz, "Pathogenesis of thoracic and abdominal aortic aneurysms.," *Ann. N. Y. Acad. Sci.*, vol. 1085, pp. 339–52, Nov. 2006.

[5] Y. Li, Z. Hu, C. Bai, J. Liu, T. Zhang, Y. Ge, S. Luan, and W. Guo, "Fenestrated and chimney technique for juxtarenal aortic aneurysm: a systematic review and pooled data analysis.," *Sci. Rep.*, vol. 6, no. February, p. 20497, 2016.

[6] M. Brand, I. Avrahami, A. Nardi, D. Silverberg, and M. Halak, "Clinical, hemodynamical and mechanical aspects of aortic aneurisms and endovascular repair," in *Aortic Aneurysms: Risk Factors, Diagnosis, Surgery and Repair*, F. Daniel and F. Hatig, Eds. New York: Nova Science Publishers Inc., 2013, pp. 181–192.

[7] I. Avrahami, M. Brand, T. Meirson, Z. Ovadia-Blechman, and M. Halak, "Hemodynamic and mechanical aspects of fenestrated endografts for treatment of Abdominal Aortic Aneurysm," *Eur. J. Mech. – B/Fluids*, vol. 35, pp. 85–91, 2012.

[8] J. E. Moore, D. N. Ku, C. K. Zarins, and S. Glagov, "Pulsatile flow visualization in the abdominal aorta under differing physiologic conditions: implications for increased susceptibility to atherosclerosis," *J. Biomech. Eng.*, vol. 114, pp. 391–397, 1992.

[9] B. Ene-Iordache, L. Mosconi, G. Remuzzi, and A. Remuzzi, "Computational fluid dynamics of a vascular access case for hemodialysis.," *J. Biomech. Eng.*, vol. 123, no. 3, pp. 284–292, 2001.

[10] F. Pecoraro, T. Pfammatter, M. Lachat, D. Mayer, Z. Rancic, M. Glenck, G. Puippe, and F. J. Veith, "Limitations to EVAR with chimney and periscope grafts," *Endovasc. Today*, no. February, pp. 56–62, 2014.

[11] G. Mestres, J. P. Uribe, C. García-Madrid, E. Miret, X. Alomar, M. Burrell, and V. Riambau, "The best conditions for parallel stenting during EVAR: an in vitro study.," *Eur. J. Vasc. Endovasc. Surg.*, vol. 44, no. 5, pp. 468–473, Nov. 2012.

[12] R. Coscas, H. Kobeiter, P. Desgranges, and J.P. Becquemin, "Technical aspects, current indications, and results of chimney grafts for juxtarenal aortic aneurysms.," *J. Vasc. Surg.*, vol. 53, no. 6, pp. 1520–1527, 2011.

[13] J. L. de Bruin, K. K. Yeung, W. W. Niepoth, R. J. Lely, Q. Cheung, A. de Vries, and J. D. Blankensteijn, "Geometric study of various chimney graft configurations in an in vitro juxtarenal aneurysm model.," *J. Endovasc. Ther.*, vol. 20, no. 2, pp. 184–190, 2013.

[14] L. Morris, P. Delassus, M. Walsh, and T. McGloughlin, "A mathematical model to predict the in vivo pulsatile drag forces acting on bifurcated stent grafts used in endovascular treatment of abdominal aortic aneurysms (AAA).," *J. Biomech.*, vol. 37, no. 7, pp. 1087–1095, 2004.

[15] T. Shipkowitz, V. G. J. Rodgers, L. J. Frazin, and K. B. Chandran, "Numerical study on the effect of steady axial flow development in the human aorta on local shear stresses in abdominal aortic branches," *J. Biomech.*, vol. 31, pp. 995–1007, 1998.

[16] G. M. H. and F. F. M. M. H. Friedman, C. B. Bargeron, D. D. Duncan, "Effects of arterial compliance and non-Newtonian rheology on correlations between intimal thickness and wall shear," *J. Biomech. Eng.*, vol. 114, no. 3, p. 317, 1992.

[17] C. A. Taylor, T. J. R. Hughes, and C. K. Zarins, "Finite element modeling of three-dimensional pulsatile flow in the abdominal aorta: relevance to atherosclerosis," *Ann. Biomed. Eng.*, vol. 26, pp. 975–987, 1998.

[18] B. T. Tang, C. P. Cheng, M. T. Draney, N. M. Wilson, P. S. Tsao, R. J. Herfkens, and C. A. Taylor, "Abdominal aortic hemodynamics in young healthy adults at rest and during lower limb exercise: quantification using image-based computer modeling.," *Am. J. Physiol. Heart Circ. Physiol.*, vol. 291, no. 2, pp. H668–H676, 2006.

[19] C. P. Cheng, R. J. Herfkens, and C. A. Taylor, "Abdominal aortic hemodynamic conditions in healthy subjects aged 50-70 at rest and during lower limb exercise: in vivo quantification using MRI," *Atherosclerosis*, vol. 168, no. 2, pp. 323–331, 2003.

[20] R. A. Jamison, G. J. Sheard, A. Fouras, and K. Ryan, "The validity of axisymmetric assumptions when investigating pulsatile biological flows," *Austral. Math. Soc.*, vol. 50, pp. 713–728, 2009.

[21] P. Tazraei, A. Riasi, and B. Takabi, "The influence of the non-Newtonian properties of blood on blood-hammer through the posterior cerebral artery," *Math. Biosci.*, vol. 264, no. 1, pp. 119–127, 2015.

[22] J. E. Moore, S. Glagovb, and D. N. Ku, "Fluid wall shear stress measurements in a model of the human abdominal aorta: oscillatory behavior and relationship to atherosclerosis," *Atherosclerosis*, vol. 9150, pp. 225–240, 1994.

[23] M. Bozzetto, B. Ene-Iordache, and A. Remuzzi, "Transitional flow in the venous side of patient-specific arteriovenous fistulae for hemodialysis," *Ann. Biomed. Eng.*, vol. 44, no. 8, pp. 2388–2401, 2016.

[24] D. N. Ku, "Blood flow in arteries," *Annu. Rev. Fluid Mech.*, vol. 29, no. 1, pp. 399–434, 1997.

[25] Y. Li, T. Zhang, W. Guo, C. Duan, R. Wei, Y. Ge, X. Jia, and X. Liu, "Endovascular chimney technique for juxtarenal abdominal aortic aneurysm: a systematic review using pooled analysis and meta-analysis," *Ann. Vasc. Surg.*, vol. 29, no. 6, pp. 1141–1150, 2015.